herbal
folk
medicine

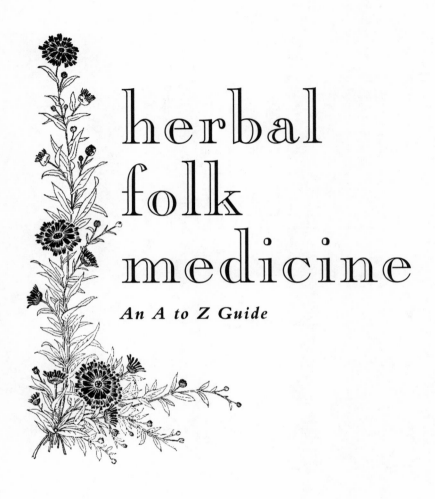

herbal
folk
medicine

An A to Z Guide

Thomas Broken Bear Squier
with Lauren David Peden

AN OWL BOOK

Henry Holt and Company   New York

This book is intended as a general guide. The authors and publisher make no claims or warranties as to the effectiveness of treatments described herein and disclaim any liability arising out of anyone's misuse of, or undue reliance on, any information provided in this book.

Henry Holt and Company, Inc.
Publishers since 1866
115 West 18th Street
New York, New York 10011

Henry Holt ® is a registered
trademark of Henry Holt and Company, Inc.

Copyright © 1997 by Thomas Squier
All rights reserved.
Published in Canada by Fitzhenry & Whiteside Ltd.,
195 Allstate Parkway, Markham, Ontario L3R 4T8.

Library of Congress Cataloging-in-Publication Data
Squier, Thomas K.
    Herbal folk medicine : an a to z guide / Thomas Broken Bear Squier
    with Lauren David Peden.
        p.   cm.
    "An Owl book."
    Includes bibliographical references.
    ISBN 0-8050-3724-1 (pb : alk. paper)
        1. Herbs—Therapeutic use—Encyclopedias.   I. Peden, Lauren
    David.   II. Title.
    RM666.H33S686   1998
    615'.321'03—dc21   97-27236

Henry Holt books are available for special
promotions and premiums. For details contact:
Director, Special Markets.

First edition 1997

Designed by Paula R. Szafranski

Printed in the United States of America
All first editions are printed on acid-free paper. ∞

10   9   8   7   6   5   4   3   2   1

This book is
lovingly dedicated
to my mother,
Helen Rebecca Jones Squier,
and
our friends at
Hoke County Hospice,
St. Joseph's of the Pines.

I cannot begin
to thank enough my wife,
Frances,
for her support and encouragement,
and my agent,
Victoria Sanders,
for her faith in me.

Contents

Preface

The Country Doctor's Legacy

More than ever before, Americans are showing an interest in using herbs and botanical preparations for treating injuries and ailments. Some attribute this to the skyrocketing cost of medical care and prescription drugs. Some are concerned about the side effects of the chemicals in many medications and the way they interact in our bodies. And still others want to be less reliant upon physicians and more in control of their own health care.

Many people are also becoming part of a back-to-the-earth movement, which involves using natural fibers, eating healthier foods, recycling, and practicing natural or alternative healing methods, in particular herbal medicine. Regardless of the specific reason for Americans' growing interest in homeopathic (natural) remedies, one thing is certain: our interest in alternative medical treatments isn't so much *new* as it is *renewed*, because we have plenty of information with

Preface

which to quench our intellectual thirst, thanks in large part to our multicultural ancestors. We are fortunate in this country to have the greatest storehouse of botanical and herbal medical knowledge in the world, and that knowledge is the country doctor's legacy.

One of the most widely used clichés concerning America is that it is a "melting pot" in which different cultures contribute their historical knowledge and unique characteristics for the good of all. With the possible exception of the dinner table, nowhere is this more visible than in herbal medicine, as developed by the country doctor of nineteenth-century America and as practiced today. Novels and journals, television dramas and films, all portray the country doctor as an important person in the American frontier community and also one of the most highly respected. Thirty years ago, Doc Adams was a beloved character on the television serial *Gunsmoke*, despite his cantankerous nature. He frequently turned to the Indians for their medical knowledge, and Marshall Dillon was saved a time or two when the Indians cured fevers and infections with mysterious herbs they had collected. The current television program *Dr. Quinn, Medicine Woman* offers another testimony to the way the country doctor learned to use the herbal treatments of the Native Americans.

In traveling across the country, one can always find herbs woven into the tapestry of our history. Whether touring the Malcolm Blue homesite in Aberdeen, North Carolina; the preserved and restored homes and shops of Plymouth and Salem, Massachusetts; Old Salem, North Carolina; or the missions of the Southwest—one will always find the herb garden portrayed as an essential part of local life. George Washington's and Thomas Jefferson's interest in natural medicines is chronicled in their papers and recreated in the gardens so carefully maintained today for visitors to their estates.

At the Elizabethan Gardens on the Outer Banks of North Carolina, one can see wonderful examples of the medicinal herbal gardens grown by the English settlers. At the Alamo in San Antonio, there is an herb garden with a special section emphasizing various forms of cayenne peppers. The National Botanical Garden in our nation's capital has a section devoted to healing herbs.

The Oconaluftee Cherokee village on the Qualla Reservation in the mountains of North Carolina, a living museum, has an herb garden for display, as well as to provide herbs for the treatment of today's illnesses and ailments. The same is true of Chucalissa Indian Village in Memphis and the restored ruins of the Anasazi Indians in Mesa Verde, Colorado. Off the coast of South Carolina there are island villages where the people have maintained much of their African heritage. Here, healers use the knowledge passed down through the generations to grow and gather herbs for healing the sick. More than any other aspect of American history, herbal medicine is truly the melting pot of America.

In the small town of Bailey, North Carolina, is the Museum of the Country Doctor, the horseback- and buggy-riding healer of the frontier and the turn-of-the-century era. On display is the legacy of these country doctors—a truly eclectic body of healing knowledge not found in other countries whose native and natural healing techniques were limited by history, geography, and warfare.

Some early country doctors certainly shared a common heritage of having received formal medical training in Europe, usually Paris, London, or Vienna. Other practitioners, particularly on the frontier following the Civil War, were untrained people who became doctors because the demand was so high for anyone with even a rudimentary knowledge of medicine. In frontier America, they learned herbal treatments, a healing approach that was just as important as European methods such as bloodletting, applying leeches, or administering metallic salts, and frequently safer and more effective. A great deal of this herbal instruction was supplemented by the Bible, which contains hundreds of references to various plants and herbs for healing. The physician who emigrated to America often had a strong religious background and a wide knowledge of plants as medicines. Some of these physicians became America's country doctors.

The harsh conditions of pioneer life created new challenges for Europe-educated physicians, which led them to adopt indigenous practices. The greatest influence on the eclectic knowledge base of these country doctors was undoubtedly the Indian medicine man, who used native botanical treatments culled from thousands of years of experimentation and knowledge.

There is really no such field as general Indian medicine, Indian culture, or even Indian cuisine. Native Americans were a large collection of separate and distinct tribes and nations, each with its own medical and cultural practices. Native Americans in one part of the country were often completely unaware of the Native Americans in a distant part of this same continent.

The Europe-trained medical personnel who became the country doctors changed all that. They not only learned the plants and healing methods of Native Americans wherever they went, but they also gleaned from their fellow immigrants the medical knowledge of their particular cultures. Country doctors learned to use the herbs and healing methods of Chinese railroad builders, of African and Middle Eastern slaves and their traders, and of the people of India, South America, and the Caribbean, where European domination was also occurring. Today, eliminating the mythical and mystical parts of the equation and taking advantage of what science can teach us about the components and properties of these plants is the responsibility of the modern herbalist.

Who can doubt that herbs and other plants will continue to be the source of new discoveries and developments in medical science for many years to come? Look at the example of Taxol, a drug derived from the yew tree that has successfully battled ovarian cancer. We still have not been able to duplicate this drug in the laboratory. Who can doubt that herbal medicine will continue to flourish in popularity in the near future and over the long haul? Perhaps the effective use of herbs for centuries will become as accepted as tests imposed by government agencies in assessing the safety and efficacy of herbal medicine and other forms of alternative healing. The chart which follows shows the long history of using plants for healing.

In this country, it is impossible to think about herbal medicine without thinking about politics. Daniel B. Mowrey has come to be looked on as something of the devil's advocate: in his books on herbal medicine he verifies some actual benefits and destroys long-held beliefs about what a particular herb will or won't do. In *The Scientific Validation of Herbal Medicine,* he writes, "Medical science in America is a unique combination of economic and political factors, which fuse together almost religiously to promote synthesized, highly active chemicals which have been around a whole ten to fifteen years. Interesting criteria are used to select which chemicals to promote. Efficacy is, of course, a necessary condition. But it is not sufficient. The chemical must be potentially profitable. Medicines that cannot be patented (or otherwise made proprietary) are not economically acceptable." He hits the nail squarely on the head with this observation: "No matter how good a substance is, if a particular pharmaceutical firm does not have the inside track on patent rights, or if such rights are unobtainable, that firm is not going to invest millions of dollars into research and marketing." For a rounded view of pharmaceutical firms, which often devote as much energy to profit as they do to research, this next statement of Dr. Mowrey's is even more telling. "If users of a natural, unpatentable, product represent an attractive market share, competitive marketing practices demand that the natural product be discredited, and its users converted to a patented, synthesized product."

Pharmaceutical firms are lobbying to have all food supplements, herbs sold in health stores, vitamins, and any similar products regulated by the FDA and made available only by prescription from licensed medical doctors. These firms have justifiably garnered a lot of atten-

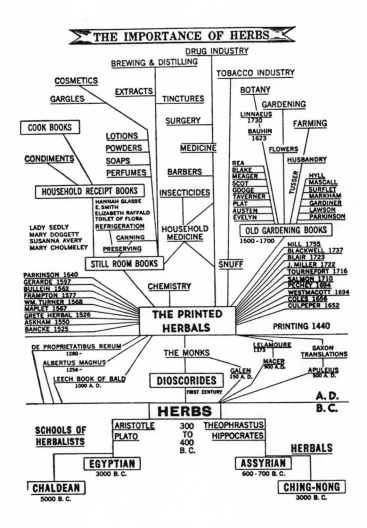

The Importance of Herbs.

Courtesy Karen Park Jennings,
senior vice president, Park Seed Company.

tion in the media and the halls of politics. Every major pharmaceutical firm is looking into dozens of herbs so they can promote them, but only after they have been altered to the point of being patentable and, by extension, marketable.

Even herbalists have begun to censor themselves because of the drug companies' hype surrounding "unproven" herbal remedies. One very knowledgeable and reputable teacher of herbal medicine sent me a list of plants she uses and teaches about with an apology: "I am sorry, but these aren't proven remedies. They have always worked for us, so maybe they will be of some use to you." But my files are filled with letters from people who use certain herbs for medicines with great success.

My own grandfather, a Cherokee "root doctor," taught me much of what I know about using plants for medicine. He was definitely a healer. He had a knowledge of what plants would work in which conditions, but because he was not a formally educated man he would today be looked upon as primitive. He may have been illiterate, but the hands-on knowledge he had about plants would fill volumes. Some pharmaceutical firms use the same plants he did, but disguise their natural origins by using their scientific names. For instance, one drug for joint pain is now being promoted on television as containing "the ingredient most prescribed by doctors." That ingredient is capsaicin, the scientific name for the active ingredient in ground-up red pepper, which my grandfather used quite effectively to treat the same pain.

I can make natural aspirin from the bark of various trees. Pharmaceutical firms will tell you that you can overdose on this natural aspirin. You can, I admit. The symptom? Tinnitus—or ringing in the ear. However, this problem, brought on by drinking too much natural aspirin tea, quickly goes away as the body metabolizes the salicylic acid. Store-bought, so-called "safe" aspirin, on the other hand, can create problems with blood clotting and may cause bleeding ulcers, perforated intestines, and other stomach problems, as well as Reye's syndrome in children. For some reason, though, you never find pharmaceutical companies publicizing these unwanted side effects. I wonder why not?

There are thousands of other herbal remedies besides aspirin that would put the drug companies out of business if they ever caught on big with the general public. To relieve congestion in my chest, I boil eucalyptus leaves in a pan and inhale the steam in a process called inhalation therapy. It works, but is denounced as "witch doctor medicine" by doctors who would rather charge you for an office visit, tell you to buy a vaporizer [humidifier or mister], and write you a prescription for eucalyptol under some other name or suggest an over-the-counter form such as Vicks VapoRub. The examples are practically limitless.

In fact, natural medicines—mostly derived from herbs—are a primary source of medicine in some 80 percent of the world. The United States joins with other nations in sending emissaries around the globe both to study herbal medicine and to tell the indigenous peoples which of their own plants Western scientists believe will heal sicknesses.

The irony, of course, is that while public relations specialists representing pharmaceutical companies deride the native healers and their practices as primitive, they are simultaneously seeking to learn these healers' secrets. Even when studying the highly developed Asian cultures, these Western specialists dismiss the practice of seeking out herbs—or synthetic medicines, for that matter—that can cure more than one disease or condition. For me, there is a very good explanation for the establishment's resistance to this holistic approach: the profit margin. Our pharmaceutical industry promotes using one drug for one condition. One drug for one illness makes for many more drug sales, bulging medicine cabinets, and greater profits. And oftentimes the underlying condition is not corrected, meaning that more drugs are sold, masking symptoms without really healing.

Preface

In the latest *Nutrition Desk Reference,* the authors, Robert Garrison, Jr., and Elizabeth Somer, who are registered pharmacists, make this statement: "From 1960 to 1995, the cost of health care in the United States escalated from $27 billion to more than $600 billion, a more than 22-fold increase. This after-the fact treatment approach to disease has not resulted in substantial improvements in the nation's health. A preventive approach, which includes individual responsibility for changing life-threatening habits, must be encouraged." Preventive medicine, including herbal treatments, is much cheaper and healthier than after-the-fact remedies.

Here is some food for thought: bypass surgery for a heart condition costs a minimum of $40,000 these days, whereas a year of diet and lifestyle therapy costs around $6,000. Of course, in the case of bypass surgery time may be of the essence. Even in less threatening conditions, though, the cost differences are comparable. The drug Ceclor would cost around $65 for a full course of treatment of an inner-ear infection, whereas an equally effective treatment of warm garlic oil would cost under $4. For a migraine headache the injection of D.H.E. 45, a popular treatment, would cost $10.26 each time the drug was administered (not counting doctor's fees and office visit charges), whereas a 30-capsule bottle of *Ginkgo biloba* extract would run around $10 and would be enough for several treatments. Except for a few rare stomach upsets, there have been no noted side effects for this treatment. Historically, chewing the leaves of feverfew herb has also proved to be a useful treatment against debilitating migraine headaches.

The high cost of pharmaceutical drugs does not all go strictly to profit, however. It currently costs around $100 million (and takes about 11 years) to get a new synthetic drug approved by the FDA and then get it patented, which allows 17 years of protected sole-production rights. A drug company has to spend just as much money and time to get the natural leaves or juice of an herb approved, but in accordance with federal regulations, it cannot patent anything that comes *directly* from a plant. It is understandable, then, why drug companies don't pursue this avenue. We must bridge this gap between nature and modern medicine by studying and documenting the effects—good and bad—of the herbs we use. Herbalists must become just as accurate and scientific in our techniques and record keeping as our pharmaceutical-company counterparts. The key is to educate ourselves to both the benefits and dangers of herbal medicines.

To derive the greatest advantage from America's herbal folk tradition, it is best to put politics aside and concentrate on seeking the information you need to improve and maintain your health safely and economically. Herbalists will never put the drug companies out of business. We shouldn't and we can't. Instead, we must concentrate on sharing accurate information about herbal remedies and policing our own ranks to prevent the dissemination of inaccurate or dangerous information.

Through a painstaking process of trial and error, the country doctor learned to combine the various healing traditions found in this country into an effective system, one that has been successfully used to treat a wide range of injuries and ailments. Today, we are the lucky beneficiaries of this hard-won knowledge, and it is up to each of us to make the best use of herbs and botanical preparations for better health and well-being.

herbal
folk
medicine

Introduction

As I discussed in the preface, herbal medicine is nothing new. Native healers have used plants and other natural remedies to improve the physical and mental health of their patients since before recorded history. Today, according to various authorities, some 60 percent of all the medicines we have either come directly from plants or else are synthesized botanical formulas. Still other herbs and plants are effective medicines just as they come from nature, alone or in combination with other products.

Unfortunately, American culture has gotten to the point where we expect all our medicines to provide instant relief, and television and magazine ads tell us that these expectations are realistic. The problem is that many medicines that seem to provide instant relief do little more than mask symptoms, and they do nothing to make us genuinely well or to alleviate the underlying condition that produced the symptoms in the first place. This is true whether we are talking about a prescription drug from a pharmacy, an over-the-counter medication, or an herbal preparation.

Herbs can't cure every disease or ailment, but they can help the natural healing process in almost every sickness or injury. That said, it's still important to remember that neither this book, nor any single book, can provide answers to all your questions about herbal medicine. That is a key point. When lecturing on herbal medicine, I am frequently asked, "Can you recommend one book that has the best answers and information about using plants for healing?" My reply is always the same: "No!" To be truly effective, one needs three or more points of view, especially when dealing with herbs that work quickly or on the central nervous system. Herbs are effective for a variety of conditions, and now many doctors and their patients want to know about their value as a treatment option that complements conventional medicine. With so many complicated new diseases and conditions being diagnosed today, it is probably dangerous to treat some forms of illness with herbs alone. The key is to get all the information you can about both traditional and alternative forms of treatment, and then use that knowledge to make intelligent health-care decisions.

This book is not intended as a substitute for a doctor's visit when you are sick or injured. Rather, it is intended to make the reader aware that herbs might be helpful as a medicine in their own right, or as an adjunct treatment to aid in healing an underlying condition. Federal law and many state laws make it illegal for me to tell you something like "You can settle an upset stomach with mint tea," or "Jewelweed will relieve a poison ivy rash," or "Willow bark tea is good for a headache." Penalties for making such a statement can result in fines and even time in jail. As has happened to others, if I sell vitamins unapproved by the FDA, I could become the target of a drug task force and have my doors smashed down and my employees terrorized. The material chosen for this guide includes only herbs that have been used historically and have been proved by science to contain ingredients that are effective and have no side effects. I also alert you to those that have potentially dangerous side effects. For instance, doctors still use digitalis, from the foxglove plant, to treat certain cardiac conditions because no synthesized drug can be made that does the job of this plant product. A little too much can be deadly, however, and it is hard to measure the active ingredient in any plant, especially for the herbalist who grows or collects the plants he or she uses. So it is unwise to experiment with digitalis or use it without medical supervision.

A little knowledge about herbal medicine can be like a lesson or two in karate—just enough to get you in trouble. This book introduces some 300 herbs and provides information on which ailment they have been used to treat, how to collect or harvest them, and in what form they have been used effectively. You could look at this information as a record of a part of history that is rapidly being lost, as a companion to what your doctor tells you, or as an exploration into the world of natural healing.

I have structured this book in a reader-friendly format that you should find easy to use. The opening chapter, "Herb Garden Basics," offers advice on designing and cultivating an herb garden, should you be inclined to do so. Next I give you some tips on "Herb Harvesting and Gathering," followed by a brief "Lesson in Botany." In "Herbal Preparations" I explain the various types of preparations and give step-by-step instructions for making them: infusions, decoctions, salves, syrups, elixirs, tinctures, and ointments, among other things. This is followed by the most important section of the book, the A to Z listing of the herbs themselves. For each plant you will find the plant's Latin name, its history, and a description of its medicinal properties and traditional uses. Some sections include a recipe for making a specific preparation from that herb.

Following the A to Z section are a glossary of commonly used terms, an appendix called "Ailments" (Appendix A), a resource section (Appendix B), and a bibliography. If you are seeking a remedy for a specific health problem, look it up in the "Ailments" appendix to find out what herb(s) have been used to treat that specific condition, then go back and read the herb's entry in the A to Z section to learn what type of treatment is traditionally prepared. Appendix B, "Resources," provides additional reading and reference information for those who would like to learn more about the practice of working with herbs.

As you read *Herbal Folk Medicine*, remember that I am not giving you medical advice per se. I am simply providing you with another angle to think about, some alternatives to ask your doctor about, and some choices to consider if you are a doctor, an herbalist, or a layperson concerned about the costs and side effects of synthesized drugs. This is not the final answer, but hopefully it will serve as an introduction to a new world of healing, a world that has been used successfully for thousands of years.

Herb Garden Basics

An experienced herbalist knows that it is impossible to grow all the herbs that he or she needs. For one thing, they just won't all thrive in the same habitat or climate. It would also require a tremendous amount of time to tend properly to an herb garden that could produce all the herbs one needed. Nevertheless, with the right approach and realistic expectations, one can gain true satisfaction out of an herb garden of any size, whether a quarter acre or a couple of pots on the fire escape of your city apartment.

You can grow herbs with two approaches. You can either carefully research and select the herbs that will grow in the available environment, or you can select the herbs you want to grow and alter the environment to meet their needs. The first approach is easier in that you are preselecting herbs that will assuredly thrive in the preexisting environment without the use of chemicals or special measures. The second approach requires more effort on the part of the gardener, as you will most likely need to install and maintain an artificial climate or habitat to ensure that your herbs grow and flourish. Just as for folk herbalists of yore, it may require a little trial and error in the garden to discover which herbs grow best in your climate and environment, taking into account soil, water, nutrients, sunlight, seasonal temperature extremes, and rainfall—and a host of other factors.

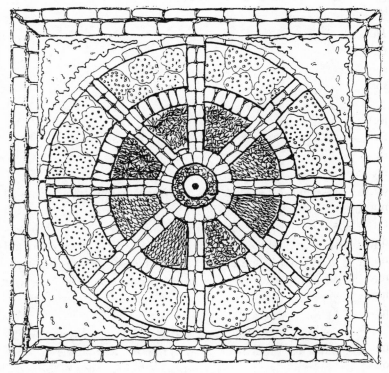

You can use a traditional herbal garden layout like this one, found at the Museum of the Country Doctor in Bailey, North Carolina, or design one to suit your own particular needs.

Herb Garden Basics

When considering the design of your herb garden, you can consult any number of books that concentrate on formal garden design, providing schematics for you to follow and all the details of construction. On the other hand, you can follow a more individual approach: sketch out your available area and plan for the spaces you already have. Many novices make the mistake of not taking into account the future shape or size of the plants or changes in available light and moisture caused by the normal growth of neighboring trees and other plants. There are numerous books on garden design, such as *Park's Success with Herbs,* and garden design computer programs, which can provide the neophyte gardener with all sorts of helpful information. Local garden shops or agricultural extension agents are usually more than willing to share their expertise, as well.

There are some general guidelines for successfully growing the majority of plants that gardeners think of as herbs: they require at least five hours of sunlight daily and require one to four inches of rainfall each month. Herbs in general do not like acidic soils—which may mean lime must be added—and they like deep, well-drained soils that do not allow water to stand or the ground to remain soggy. Herbs do not like "wet feet," so raised beds may be needed for their cultivation. Other herbs may need bog (wet) environments for growth, and if you don't have these conditions they will have to be created. Since it's just not possible to grow *every* herb that you will want to use or will need, many practicing herbalists find that it is much easier to focus on growing certain herbs, and for the rest, to collect wild plants, obtain them from reputable wildcrafters, or purchase them from supply houses.

If you don't have a lot of gardening experience, I would recommend that you plan for the space you have and begin growing herbs on a small scale. Some can be grown from seed, while others have to be propagated from cuttings or transplanted. Always be aware of an herb's native environment. Many plants have a symbiotic relationship with other plants that must be duplicated if they are to be grown successfully. After you are successful with a few basic herbs, then experiment and expand your garden.

It is very likely that you will still end up as either an herbalist or an herb gardener, but not both, because each is a full-time job (or a very time-consuming hobby). Many herbalists have a garden to relax in, and it just happens to produce some of the herbs that they need in preparing herbal remedies. And it is good to grow some of the herbs you use, especially to demonstrate or teach with.

Herb Harvesting
and Gathering

The healing properties of herbs are all subject to the vagaries of the climate, soil, sunlight, and other environmental factors. Under the best of circumstances, these factors make it difficult to determine the amount of active component a specific plant or part of a plant contains. One way to maximize the healing qualities is to be very familiar with the factors over which we have the most control, which include the time and season of harvest, preparation and preservation methods, and storage methods. You should also be very familiar with any area from which you intend to harvest plants. Nearby dump sites as well as chemical runoff from farmland or highways, and other man-made pollutants, may render plants from these spots unusable.

Herbs should be collected or harvested when, to the best of our knowledge, the active components are at their maximum levels. We can't just set this time by the calendar. We must be familiar with the plant we are harvesting and the conditions under which it has been growing. Hard winters, late springs, or early springs can have effects on plants that we must learn either to take advantage of or to overcome.

Being aware of a plant's life cycle can also be very valuable. Perennial plants and trees go through a cycle of activity and dormancy. For example, even though we can harvest sassafras roots all year round, they are most potent when gathered during the winter, the period when the sap is "down." Annuals or biennials go through a cycle of growth and death during which the plant has a definitive "effective" period. For example, it is important to know that with a plant like the wild carrot, which lives two years, the root is most powerful in the first winter when the most food is stored and the plant is preparing for the coming season of blooming and seed production.

In addition to knowing about a plant's life cycle, it's also important to familiarize yourself with the various parts of the plant and the procedures for collecting, storing, and using them. Subterranean parts, roots and rhizomes, are usually dug up at the end of the vegetational season or in the fall, when the plant is preparing for the winter's "sleep." (A rhizome is a subterranean plant stem that is thickened by deposits of reserve food.) Hard, woody roots should be allowed to dry and stored in a cool, dry place. The longer they are kept whole, the longer they maintain their strength. Special care should be taken when handling fleshy roots and rhizomes, since they damage easily. Shake off the soil, which may harbor pests or destructive organisms, and allow the root to dry before storage (this applies to all roots, not just fleshy ones). Some fleshy roots, such as carrots and parsnips, are best stored where they are grown, without any handling, if used quickly thereafter. You may also store them in a root cellar or any cool, dark, dry place. Some people store root vegetables in a barrel of dry sand.

Bulbs and tubers are usually dug up in the autumn as soon as the leaves and other above-ground parts of the plant turn brown and fade back. Some plants and plant parts contain chemicals that are dangerous or should be avoided as much as possible. A plant harvester should wear protective clothing and only collect one type of plant at a time before washing her hands. Avoid eating, drinking, and smoking until the job is done to avoid contaminating plant material and/or accidentally medicating or poisoning yourself; poisonous and nonpoisonous plants should never be collected or stored together. To avoid making a potentially dangerous mistake, it is best to concentrate on one or two plant species or parts at a time. Also, avoid handling plants when you have open cuts or sores on your hands or skin, to prevent direct absorption of chemicals or irritants.

Aerial parts, parts of the plant found above ground, should be collected when they are in the best condition: when dew has evaporated and before the heat of the day has had its effect on the plants. Harvest the leaves and flowers carefully to avoid damage and store in firm containers for the same reason. Baskets are best for storage because they allow for the circulation of air.

Leaves should be collected when young but fully grown, and they should be healthy, clean, and free of debris and contaminants. Leaves are usually best collected before flowering occurs.

It is best to collect flowers at the early stage of their flowering period and during the part of day when they are free of dew but not subjected to drying winds and heat, which remove volatile oils. In many cases flowers will continue to develop after being picked. Once again, baskets are best for storage, since flowers stored in airtight containers often "sweat" and deteriorate quickly if it is very hot. You can also hang them in a dark space where air circulates freely.

Herbage, the combined leaves, stalks, and flowers together, is collected when the plant begins to flower. Avoid stalks that are too thick and the woody bases of herbaceous plants. Herbage from aquatic plants might need to be transported in some quantity of water to prevent deterioration, which can occur quickly once the plant begins to dry out.

Bark is collected in the spring when the flow of sap is at its peak and its active principles are most powerful. Make parallel cuts up and down the branch that the plant can heal over and lift off portions of bark. Do not girdle a tree or shrub to obtain bark, as this will kill the plant (girdling is a technique that removes the tree's bark in one continuous circle). Naturally you should take care not to kill any trees when you gather herbs; not only is it ecologically unsound, but it will work against you later. A dead tree cannot be used as an herb source in the future.

When wood of a plant is called for, it refers to a large branch or a small trunk that can be cut into manageable pieces. Wood is probably the least-used part of plants for medicinal purposes; it is more suited to smoking foods and adding flavor in preservation.

Fruit is collected when it begins to ripen because the process of ripening will also continue after it is harvested. Seeds are removed from mature fruit and if the seed is the desired part, any fleshy covering is removed to prevent spoilage or, in some cases, germination.

Herbs are dried and stored in different manners according to their consistency. The key to drying herbs is to eliminate the damaging effects of heat and light as much as possible, but attention should also be given to the plant's water content. The parts with the most liquid in them require the most effort to preserve. Drying consists of removing as much of the water as possible from the tissues. Special attention should be given to the distinct drying requirements of each plant and each part of the plant. It takes about one square yard of open space to dry one pound of flowers because they must be spread out, not touching, to allow maximum circulation of air. Many leaves, on the other hand, can be dried between layers of stacked newspapers (as long as they're printed with soy or other nontoxic ink).

Large woody plants can be hung in bunches upside down and stored in a dark place where the air moves freely. Fleshy plants require different treatment. Rather than try to preserve the plant whole, it might be better to cut it in smaller pieces and freeze them or place them in oil or alcohol to extract their properties.

A drying apparatus is available commercially, but it is also easy to make one. Screen or hardware cloth makes for an effective drying rack. Larger parts of the plant should be observed during the drying process and turned to prevent spoilage and mildew and to permit even drying. Fruits can be cut up and sun-dried or dried over a low-level heat source with a free exchange of air, such as an oven on very low heat, with the door kept ajar to permit moisture to escape. You want the plant to dry, not cook!

Roots should be arranged without touching each other until completely dry and then handled carefully to avoid breaking.

Do not dry or store different plants or plant parts together, and be certain to carefully label and date all materials and the different storage containers. You also might want to record where the plants came from in the event that problems arise later.

A Lesson in Botany

Every herbalist needs some working knowledge of the active part of the plants he or she uses. Students of botany spend an entire semester or more learning all the parts of plants, so we won't fool ourselves into thinking that we are going to be botanists after reading this brief section. However, a quick lesson will get you started on the right foot. The more you know about the structure of plants, the easier it will be to comprehend other sources of information, and the easier it will be to work with materials, remedies, and people.

The plants we are concerned with for the most part have four basic parts: the root, the stem, the leaf, and the flower or fruit. In most cases, the flower is the part that becomes the fruit. Some plants have flowers with both male and female components, and these plants are called self-pollinating. Even so, usually the male parts from one flower pollinate the female parts from another flower. Other plants have separate male and female flowers; sometimes they are found on the same plant, and sometimes on separate male and female plants. In that case, you will need both male and female plants in order for them to bear fruit. Some plants are controlled by having only either male or female specimens. The ginkgo, for example, is usually sold only as female in this country without the males necessary to ensure fruit production. This prevents the formation of fruit, which has an offensive smell.

The male reproductive parts of a flower are called the stamens, and the female part is the pistil; the pistil is made up of the ovary, the style, and the stigma.

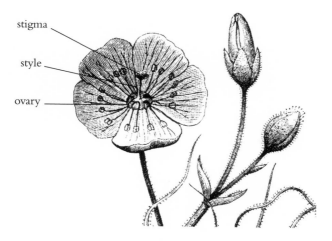

stigma
style
ovary

Female parts of a flower.

The stem supports the plant and transports nutrients from the roots to the leaves and flowers. A rhizome is considered to be a root by many, but it is actually a special type of stem designed to store reserves of food for the plant's future needs. Rhizomes usually lie just under the surface of the soil.

In most cases, the root is the part of the plant that anchors it to the soil. Roots can take different shapes, depending on whether they will have to store foods over the winter or during a dormant period. Tap-

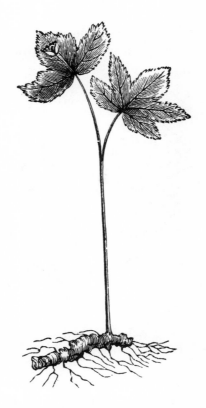

A rhizome is actually an enlarged underground stem.

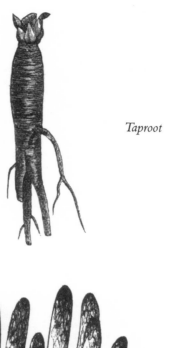

Taproot

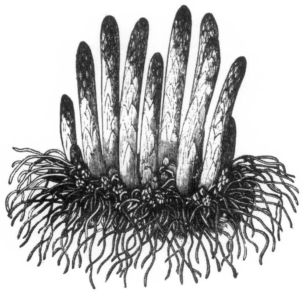

The moplike root of an asparagus plant is called a crown.

19

roots dig deep to bring up minerals and nutrients, while the moplike roots of asparagus serve as a solid base for the top-heavy mature plant. Roots can also have special structures, such as tubers—potatoes, dahlias, and begonias grow from tubers—which store foods or permit asexual reproduction.

In most green flowering plants, the leaf is the structure where photosynthesis occurs. For the herbalist, a leaf is a leaf. However, in identifying plants in the field, it is important to know something about leaf shape or form and the type of edge the leaf characteristically

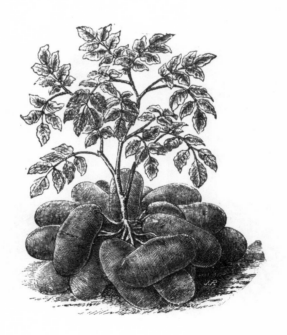

Potatoes are tubers.

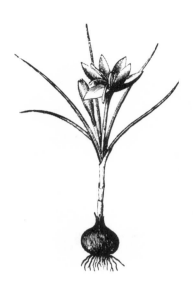

The bulbs of onions and other similar plants store food below ground.

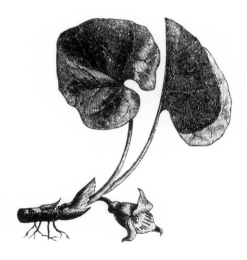

A smooth, lobed leaf. In this case, the heart-shaped leaf of wild ginger.

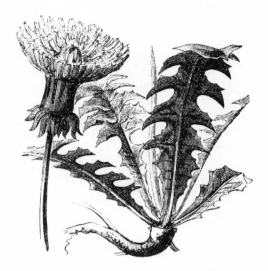

A toothed leaf. In this case, the leaf of the dandelion.

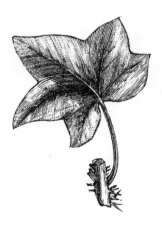

A lobed leaf. In this case, an ivy leaf.

displays—smooth, toothed, lobed, serrated—because these different patterns are sometimes the only way to tell one herb from another.

A gardener, herbalist, or anyone else seriously interested in plants should become as familiar as possible with the botanical, or scientific, names of plants. They are Latin, consist of a genus name and a species name, and may be derived from Greek or Latin roots. Some words tip off the reader about the plant's use, characteristics, or appearance. For example, *luten* means yellow, *rubra* means red, *album* or *alba* means white, *stellarin* means starlike, and *vulgare* means common or widespread.

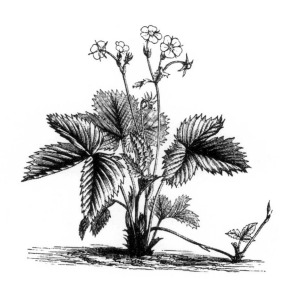

A serrated leaf. In this case, the leaf of the strawberry plant.

Herbal Preparations

The folk herbalist may be challenged by some of the techniques described below, because the equipment or technology either is not available or is too large to set up and maintain, or because the cost is prohibitive. Some distillation processes may be possible, but be aware that this is getting into a legal gray area, since alcohol is used as a solvent for oils or other substances and then distilled off from the finished product. Nonetheless, a few basic herbal preparations and techniques will be elaborated on here, because even if the herbalist can't perform them, understanding how the preparation is obtained may be useful.

Infusions and Teas

An infusion is what most people think of as a tea. An infusion is an aqueous preparation that can be taken internally or used externally as a wash, a rinse, or even a douche. Some herbalists consider it an infusion only if the end product is made from leaves, flowers, and other tender parts of the herb or plant, and not from the roots, bark, etc. Some use other parts of the plant. The key is that boiling water is poured on the herb and then it is steeped, usually covered to prevent the loss of volatile oils and other chemicals that might otherwise be lost in the steam. Older herbal books may refer to an infusion as a tisane.

With some herbs we are interested only in the water-soluble components, and these herbs may be soaked for some period of time in cold water, usually in a sealed container to prevent contamination.

The herb can be loose in the cup or other container, sealed in a tea bag or cloth bag, or held in a tea ball. Some herbalists are now making some of their infusions in "sun-tea jars," which involves placing the tea bags in water in a sealed jar and setting it in a sunny spot, thereby allowing the sun's light and heat to extract the chemicals into the water.

It is important not to confuse a genuine herbal infusion with commercially available herb teas. The latter usually contain about $\frac{1}{16}$ of an ounce of herb and are just for flavor. In herbal preparations that will be prescribed medicinally, we typically use an ounce or more of herb to one pint of water or perhaps some other proportion. These teas are definitely far more potent than the herb teas sold as sleeping aids or beverages.

Decoctions

Decoctions are similar to infusions but they are processed by boiling the water or simmering it for a longer period of time. Some herbalists consider an aqueous preparation a decoction if it is made from harder parts of herbs or plants such as bark, roots, seed pods, or other parts that require boiling to extract any active component successfully. In this case, we often start with 1½ pints of water to one ounce of herb and let it simmer down to one pint. Both decoctions and infusions are considered to be temporary preparations and are usually prepared on a daily basis or as needed and rarely stored, except for a few days under refrigeration.

A rule of thumb in making both decoctions and infusions is that about one teaspoon of herb to one pint water is used in the treatment of acute conditions and one tablespoon of herb to one quart of water in the treatment of chronic conditions. Practice and experience will begin to guide your ratios and mixtures after a little while.

Herbal Steams

Herbal steams are generally used to clear out congestion from the nasal or bronchial passages, much like an electric vaporizer with an herb added. Eucalyptus oil is used in this way to fill a closed room or tent with therapeutic vapors. Breathing deeply during the steaming process helps to increase the effectiveness of the herb, adds hydration, and breaks up mucus and phlegm. This process is also known as inhalation therapy, and can be as simple as holding a towel or other cloth over a steaming pot of herbs and placing the cloth over the nose and mouth to breathe in the steam when it is cool enough to be safe, or it may involve more sophisticated or modern equipment like the vaporizer or mister. Native Americans use inhalation therapy in their sweat lodges. By pouring a mixture of water and herbs on heated rocks, they cleanse the physical body of poisons, as well as cleanse the spirit.

Herbs commonly used for steaming include eucalyptus, thyme, rosemary for headaches, mint, mullein, and sage.

Some herbalists also use herbal steams for cosmetic purposes. One of the more popular forms is a facial steam to clear the complexion or remove impurities. Some herbs used in this manner include yarrow, lavender, rose petals, calendula, elder flowers, and lemon balm.

Infused Oils

Infused oils can be made quickly in the top of a double boiler using olive oil or other vegetable oils and the appropriate herbs. The goal is to heat the oil, not to cook it. Let the dried herbs and flowers simmer for two hours or until they're wilted but not fried, then strain. Eucalyptus oil made in this manner is an excellent decongestant when rubbed on the chest. Fresh herbs and flowers can also be used, but you must remove the water that cooks out to prevent spoilage. You also have to strain out the brownish accumulation in the bottom of the jar, which is left after you have poured off all but the last little bit.

It is also easy to make infused oils by placing the herb in olive or another oil and leaving the container in the sun or a warm area. Two to three weeks later, strain out the herb and remove excess water with a filter.

Herbal Salves and Balms

Salves and balms are applied externally to ease the pain of sores, strains, sprains, and burns (thermal or sunburn). They can be made by combining herb-infused oil with melted beeswax. Both the oils and the beeswax must be warm, and all utensils and containers must be heated and kept warm or the beeswax will begin to set on contact.

A good beeswax-to-oil proportion is 1¼ ounces of melted beeswax to one cup of herb-infused oil, but this can be adjusted with practice or according to need to make stiffer or softer salves. Ladle the oil and beeswax combination into heated jars and allow to cool with a piece of cheesecloth or wax paper on top. This will prevent debris from contaminating the salve and will also eliminate condensation, which occurs when lids are placed on too soon.

Syrups

Herbal syrups are made with juices or infusions of herbs. You can even make them from whole herbs, but these syrups must be strained for clarity and purity. Basically a syrup is made with two parts refined sugar to one part distilled water and the herbal product that you wish to use. Bring the water to a boil, add the sugar and stir to dissolve it, and then simmer. To make the syrup last longer without spoiling, it can be preserved by adding some portion of glycerine in place of the water. How much depends on the situation; it's a skill learned by experience so you may have to try a few times before hitting the correct measurement. Start by substituting glycerine for half of the water. Glycerine is available in most pharmacies.

Elixirs

Elixirs contain alcohol and water and are often labeled "cough syrups" and sold as over-the-counter and prescription medications. Many labels say that the medication contains a percentage of alcohol, so read your labels carefully. Nevertheless, since alcohol is sometimes the best solvent for certain herbs, you may find its use necessary. One formula for an elixir is to make a syrup according to the directions above and combine it with an equal part vodka. You can use other liquors, but vodka is most commonly used because it is relatively inexpensive, clear, and somewhat flavorless. Gins and whiskeys add their own flavors to the elixir. Vodka is usually either 80 proof (40 percent alcohol) or 100 proof (50 percent alcohol). The higher the alcohol content, the more the herb is dissolved or the more herb can be dissolved. But beware. It has been found, for example, that the alcohol in the elixir of cascara sagrada used as a laxative in some V.A. and military hospitals can become habit forming.

Tinctures

A tincture results when alcohol instead of water is used to extract the desired properties from herbs. A tincture is much more concentrated than an infusion, decoction, or elixir, and a little goes a long way. Often tinctures are administered under the tongue in one- or two-drop doses. Most herbalists use vodka to make their tinctures. However, some use a 95 percent alcohol product called Everclear, a powerful solvent that is extremely flammable and that, since it will dissolve Styrofoam cups and some plastics, must be stored in glass containers.

To make a tincture, steep one ounce of herb in five ounces of alcohol for six weeks. Strain and seal carefully. Keep it out of direct sunlight or bright light and shake it every two or three days. If the level of liquid diminishes during the process, replenish it. Since tinctures' potency can prove hazardous, make a special effort to keep them out of the reach of small children.

Some gums and unwanted precipitates are produced in the making of tinctures and can be strained out for clarity and appearance.

Ointments

Ointments are thicker than salves and are just as easy to make. You can mix a desired amount of tincture into a commercial ointment at a ratio of one to one or ½ ounce tincture to one ounce ointment.

You can also make your own ointment using beeswax and lard, lanolin, or natural oils such as almond, olive, or wheat-germ oil. Cocoa butter can also be used. Be aware that lanolin comes from sheep and some people are allergic to it. Some may be allergic to lard, which is rendered pork fat. It is available in grocery stores, often in five-gallon buckets. Look for the Spanish name *manteca* where there are large Latino populations.

To make the basic ointment, mix eight ounces of melted lard with two ounces melted beeswax. (Because pure beeswax can be expensive, some herbalists mix it with paraffin sealing wax, which is cheaper.) A basic herbal ointment is made by simmering the lard, lanolin, or oil with the herb for several hours on as low a heat as possible. The ointment can be made stronger by straining out the old herbs and adding new ones. Melt the wax so that the lard and the wax are the same temperature and combine, stirring well to ensure even mixing. Pour into the warmed containers the ointment will be stored in, cool, and seal.

Suppositories and Pessaries

A suppository is a small cylinder of medicated material that is inserted into a bodily cavity such as the rectum. A pessary is a vaginal suppository.

Suppositories and pessaries are made in pencil-shaped molds with one end narrower than the other so that the suppository is shaped somewhat similar to the tip of a carrot. You can make molds from aluminum foil or buy commercially available molds (molds are two inches long and half an inch in diameter). Lightly oil the molds with olive oil and place them in the freezer. Heat cocoa butter and the herb product and simmer slightly. The basic ratio is three ounces of cocoa butter to one ounce of powdered herb. Pour the melted mixture into the cold molds and shape them as necessary. When they have cooled, remove the suppositories from the molds, wrap them with cellophane or wax paper, and store them in the refrigerator or another cool place.

Witch hazel is often used to make an astringent suppository to shrink hemorrhoids.

Extracts

Extracts are made by boiling (distilling) off most of the liquid portion of fresh herbs, collecting the resultant mass, and then adding alcohol as a preservative. To get the most strength from your extract, combine the herbs with water, boil it down to a paste, add more water, and repeat. Repeat the process one more time and then add a minute amount of alcohol to preserve the herb.

Pills and Capsules

Not many herbalists make pills routinely anymore because gelatin capsules are readily available to be filled with the herbal powder. If you do want to make pills, however, combine equal amounts of herb powder and corn starch, add just enough water to make the mixture moist, and then roll the material into tiny balls. Spread them to dry and store them. For sudden needs or treatments of brief duration, you can make a pill by mixing the herb with about 1/16 teaspoon of cream cheese or firm, well-drained tofu.

Generally, it is a simple process to fill capsules with herb or herb powder, especially with bitter or other herbs that taste bad. Racks can be made that hold the bottom half of the capsule. Then add the powdered herb and seal the capsule with the other half. Store as you would other medications.

Absorbent Pads

Sterile absorbent pads can be made by boiling dried sphagnum moss, then drying it completely. The dried moss is either used directly or wrapped in cloth to make wound dressings, sanitary napkins, or diapers. Herbal preparations can be added. Garlic oil, for example, is used to fight infection, while mint helps control unpleasant odors.

Poultices

Poultices are crushed or chopped fresh herbs applied to a wound or skin problem such as hemorrhoids, swollen eyes, boils, or burns. In the case of puffy eyelids or hemorrhoids, the poultice can be as simple and as quick as applying a wet tea bag and allowing the tannin from the tea to reduce the swelling. Poultices can be applied directly as crushed herbs for such things as strains and sprains, or they can be wrapped in cloth or paper to keep messiness under control. Cold poultices are helpful in taking away heat from an area such as the site of infection or swelling, while hot poultices can promote blood flow and relax spasms. Oatmeal poultices are often applied to help with the removal of embedded foreign objects because oatmeal helps draw the offending object to the skin's surface. A poultice can also be a cloth or sphagnum moss bundle soaked with a decoction or infusion.

Plasters

Plasters are herbal powders mixed with cornstarch and applied to the affected area to provide heat, reduce swelling, or allow for absorption of the herb into the chest or other area. Mustard plasters, used for congestion and inflammation, are probably the most well known. The powdered mustard can actually burn the skin so the plaster mixture is usually wrapped in cloth. This also facilitates easy removal.

Baths and Footbaths

Cayenne pepper or some other heat-producing herb is often used in a footbath to relieve colds and flu symptoms, to promote sweating, or to relax tired feet. Herbs, usually enclosed in a cloth sack, can also be added to the bathwater to relax the bather or to provide medication to the skin. I have boiled black walnut hulls and added the resultant liquid to the bathtub to treat the family for a ringworm infestation that came along with a free cat.

Those are the basic herbal preparations. On the following pages, you will find a compendium of herbs with information on the specific uses of various plants, as well as additional instructions on how to make (and when to use) the different types of preparations.

ABSCESS ROOT. *Polemonium reptans.* Also known as American Greek Valerian in some sources, this plant was brought to America by Scandinavian seamen, who used the roots and bark in a tea for treatment of febrile conditions; it acts as a diaphoretic and an expectorant.

ACACIA GUM. *Acacia senegal.* This material came to America with the first doctors and was found in all pharmacies. Acacia gum is still used in many preparations today to soothe irritated mucous membranes, and in cough and cold remedies. Acacia gum also has been found to inhibit bacterial growth in the mouth and on the skin. It is used topically in wound-healing salves and ointments and is readily available.

Originally known as Egyptian gum because of its desert origins, where it is collected from thorny members of the legume family, acacia gum is available in the form of a gum or a powder and may be sold as gum arabic.

Acacia gum is used today in making hard candies, as it has been for centuries. It can be mixed with other herbs to form "pastilles," hard pills that dissolve slowly in the stomach—an ancient and herbal version of modern timed-release medicines. Acacia gum can be bought through pharmacies, Asian food stores, health food stores, and even hobby shops, where small bottles are sold for inclusion in chemistry sets.

Hardened acacia gum stores well, but is easily dissolved in boiling water for use as a mucilage, demulcent, and antidiarrheal. References in the Bible to shittim wood may be references to acacia.

ACEROLA CHERRY. *Malpighia glabra.* Known also as Barbados cherry, Puerto Rican cherry, or West Indian cherry, the acerola cherry came to this country early as trade with the Caribbean islands increased. It is one of the most concentrated sources of vitamin C and is used extensively as a natural vitamin C source and in the making of commercial cold medicines. The fruit is also high in vitamin A.

Eating acerola berries and drinking the juice is a treatment for scurvy and dietary deficiencies and is useful to those who take megadoses of vitamin C for the treatment and prevention of various ailments like colds and infections, as well as cancer prevention. It is emphasized that the anticancer abilities have not been proven scientifically, but many people follow a high intake of vitamin C for this purpose anyway and end up wasting money and vitamins. The human body eliminates, rather than stores, megadoses of vitamin C; a sure sign that you're taking more than you need is bright yellow or orange urine.

ADDER'S TONGUE. *Erythronium americanum.* Known more commonly today as dogtooth violet, adder's tongue is not a violet, but a lily with mottled green leaves and yellow flowers. The colonists and the Indians ate the bulbs for the calories—it is a food rich in starch; today's research also indicates some antibacterial activity. The leaves are crushed in a poultice to alleviate external ulcers; some sources say that during the Civil War, it was used to treat decubitus ulcers (bedsores) in bedridden patients. An effective poultice combines equal quantities of adder's tongue, comfrey, and plantain.

AGRIMONY. *Agrimonia eupatoria.* Called cocklebur or sticklewort, this plant is not the same cocklebur that grows in soybean fields in the South and sticks to dogs' coats. It was used to make a tea (one ounce of herb to one pint of water) taken for its antidiarrheal effect and for its effectiveness in helping with excessive flow during menstruation.

ALDER. *Alnus rugosa.* Several Indian tribes chewed the bark for toothaches as well as for cold, cough, and hives. A cold wash tea rinse made from the bark of the branches is also effective for sprains and strains when applied topically and for vaginitis and hemorrhoids as a wash. It is taken internally as a tea (one ounce of bark to one pint of water) for fever, abdominal cramps, and ulcers.

ALFALFA. *Medicago sativa.* The name comes from the Arabic *al-fasfasfah*, which means "the best fodder," but was changed to alfalfa by the Spanish. Though it didn't come to America until just before the Civil War, alfalfa quickly became popular with Native Americans. It is said to make horses run faster and cows give more milk, and herbalists use it to help humans fight conditions ranging from diabetes to alcoholism. Much of alfalfa's effectiveness is probably derived from its roots, which may extend more than 20 feet into the soil, bringing up valuable trace elements and nutrients.

ALOE VERA. *Aloe vera, A. perryi, A. barbadenis, A. vulgaris.* Most commonly known as burn plant, aloe vera is a familiar friend used for treating minor burns and other skin irritations simply by applying the crushed plant to the affected area. Aloe was carried to the New World by the Spanish in the sixteenth century and quickly became an addition to many households, often kept in the kitchen near the stove to treat burns. Aloe has been a staple in healing for centuries, being found in the Egyptian Book of Remedies dating from 1500 B.C. and long used for skin treatment and as a laxative.

Applied topically, the plant's flesh soothes burns, bedsores, insect bites, and sunburn as well as hemorrhoids.

Aloe is used in many commercial laxatives and is listed on labels as alantoin or aloe gel. A commercial preparation named Dermaide has been shown to be effective against gram-negative and -positive bacteria, thus fighting infection as a broad-spectrum antibiotic. It has also been used to treat *Candida albicans* effectively.

The dried latex of the leaves is a strong cathartic, which should be used with caution and avoided by children and those with gastric ailments. Aloe vera gel mixed with water applied topically to the affected area is a Mexican American remedy for rheumatism and arthritis.

Aloe Vera Ointment

1 tablespoon cocoa butter
2 tablespoons cornstarch
1 tablespoon aloe vera juice or gel
1,200 international units vitamin E or more (3 or more capsules)
distilled water

Form the cocoa butter into a ball and make a hole in the center. Add vitamin E oil from capsules and mix thoroughly. Work in cornstarch and aloe vera, mixing well. If it gets too stiff, add more aloe juice or gel or a little distilled water. Store in a light-proof container in a cool place.

ALUM ROOT. *Heuchera americana.* This perennial plant reaches a
height of about four feet, including the flower stalk, and grows in
shady places from Vermont southward to the mountains of Ten-
nessee, Alabama, and Arkansas and westward to Oklahoma. The
root is the predominantly used part, especially in a tea made to treat
sore throat, stomach pain, and upset stomach, and in an infusion
to treat diarrhea. The leaves were used as a poultice for sores by
many Indians and the dried leaves and roots were powdered for
the same use. Several Indian tribes used the root for treating cancers.

AMARANTH. *Amaranthus retroflexus.* One of the many plants
known as either wild spinach or pigweed, amaranth is an excellent
source of iron. With 3.9 milligrams per 100 grams, it is very effective for treating iron deficiency, especially in women. It is also high
in vitamin C, so it makes a good antiscorbutic. Indians used a poultice of amaranth for treating swellings, sprains, and aching teeth. It
is astringent, so a green tea made from amaranth is a good antidiarrheal medicine and has been used to soothe upset stomachs. The tea
made from green amaranth leaves will help stop the bleeding that
some people experience after brushing their teeth.

ANGELICA. *Angelica archangelica.* Angelica is most commonly used
as a food source and flavoring agent. It received its name because,
legend has it, angelica was revealed by an angel to humans as a cure
for the plague.

In Appalachia, the roots are gathered in the fall for winter use as
a treatment for colic and against stomach gas. A tea made from the
roots is used to control menstrual cramps and pain. The roots have
been boiled to make a breath wash and to treat sour stomach. Angelica tea has also been used to empty the stomach by causing vomiting. It has also been claimed that eating dried angelica root might
curb desire for alcohol.

The tea made from the seeds is good for treating nausea, vomiting, stomach cramps, and ulcers. The seeds are gathered when ripe and then dried, but not over a fire or in a commercial dehydrator, which tend to rob them of their strength.

Collect roots in late to middle spring for maximum effectiveness. Peel and slice thinly and dry in the sun. When crisp and completely dry, store until needed. Grind into a powder for use.

ANISE. *Pimpinella anisum.* Well known for its use in Italian cooking, anise is one of the oldest known herbs and was written about in the Bible. It has been used to increase lactation, decrease flatulence, and alleviate the cramping effect of other herbs used to stop diarrhea. A tea made from anise seed or leaves will help eliminate nausea and fight the giddiness that goes along with it in some cases.

Because of its popular licorice flavor, anise is used in making candy and in flavoring cough syrups. Women may also unconsciously find it appealing because of its slight estrogenic effect. This could explain the use of anise in aphrodisiac compounds.

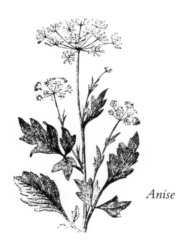

Anise

APPLE. *Malus sylvestris.* "An apple a day keeps the doctor away" is an old saying familiar to all of us. Apples came here with the colonists and are now widespread. Their fruit contains an amazing substance, pectin, which helps fight both diarrhea and constipation. In the bowels, pectin swells to form a thick, gummy mass that produces stools to stop diarrhea and also loosens compacted material in the case of constipation and lubricates the bowels to facilitate evacuation. The apple's peel is another excellent source of pectin. Pectin is the "pectate" part of the antidiarrheal commercial medication Kaopectate and is very effective.

An antibacterial substance called phloretin, found in the fruit's flesh and skin, is effective against a wide range of pathogens. The seeds of apples contain hydrogen cyanide, the poison of lethal injections, and should not be eaten.

ARBOR VITAE. *Thuja occidentalis.* The common name means "tree of life," but pregnant women should drink the tea made from the leaves with caution. A standard dose of one ounce of leaves to one pint of water acts as a diuretic and emmenagogue, but stronger doses might act as an abortifacient due to the chemicals' stimulant action on the uterus. Cedar oil, used in the drug trade, is distilled from the flattened arbor vitae leaves and is used in making both aromatic and insect-repelling soaps.

ARNICA. *Arnica montana.* Once a very popular medicinal herb among Europeans, particularly the Swiss and Germans, arnica is now recommended only as an external salve and even then should be used with caution. Old herbal texts may recommend arnica as a heart and circulatory stimulant, but one dose killed the famous Swiss naturalist Konrad Gesner after only an hour in 1565! A salve made from arnica is good for relieving pain of sore muscles, bruises, and sprains.

ARTICHOKE. *Cynara scolymus.* The flower heads of the globe artichoke are consumed as a green vegetable. All parts of the plant contain active ingredients that aid in digestion and that traditionally have been used to address complaints of a slow or sluggish liver, poor digestion and appetite, and atherosclerosis. Tea made from the leaves, roots, and flower heads has been shown to reduce blood sugars, including triglycerides, and to lower serum cholesterol levels. Two substances found in artichokes, cynarin and scolymoside, have been isolated and shown to stimulate bile secretion, which helps eliminate toxins, metabolites, and cell waste. Artichokes are also effective as diuretics.

ASH. *Fraxinus* species. A number of Indian tribes used bark from various species of ash tree brewed into a tea to treat fevers and diarrhea and kidney infections, and to reduce fever blisters. It was also used as a wash to remove the pain of sore eyes. The bark was brewed extra strong to act as an emetic and cathartic and to treat scabies and repel head lice.

ASPARAGUS. *Asparagus officinale.* This European native (see illustration on page 19) came with the colonists and has spread across the continent. Asparagus roots and stalks are used in producing diuretics. Simply drink the water produced by cooking, but beware—asparagus produces a strong odor in the urine. Raw asparagus may act as a laxative.

ASPIRIN. Aspirin is made from the bark of spirea bushes and willow trees and other plants that contain the chemical salicylic acid or salicylate. Synthetic aspirin, patented around 1893 by the Bayer company, is known as ASA or acetylsalicylic acid and does not duplicate nature's formula. The extra "acetyl" of commercial aspirin makes it more acidic, so those taking it in long-term therapy require some antacid, because the acid dissolves mucous membranes and the stomach lining, causing ulcers and internal bleeding. Pharmaceutical lobbyists warn against overdosing with willow bark and other natural aspirins because it is virtually impossible for the average person, even an herbalist, to determine the chemical content and strength of a leaf or twig. Using the standard of one ounce of herb to a pint of water, the actual amount of aspirin present could vary according to the part of the plant used, the climatic and meteorologic factors, and the time of year harvested. The symptom and problem of overdosing with natural aspirin is tinnitus, or ringing in the ears. It is relieved by either using less herb in preparation or reducing the amount of the decoction taken.

The problems associated with even recommended doses of commercial aspirin, on the other hand, can include thinned blood, which means bleeding and clotting problems following injuries or surgery, bleeding ulcers, perforated bowel, and, more rarely, Reye's syndrome, especially in children. See WILLOW.

ASTRAGALUS. *Astragalus membranaceus.* The Chinese, who call this member of the vetch family *huang ch'i*, have dried its roots for centuries and used them in the treatment of hypertension and to boost the immune system in patients suffering from cancer and other ailments. Research verifies it is effective for this and for the treatment of the degenerative disease myasthenia gravis. Astragalus can now be found growing wild in this country and is known as milk vetch, and its prepared roots can be obtained in standardized dosage extracts in health food stores. The roots are still sun-dried, and then a water–alcohol extraction process at low temperature provides a quantifiable free flowing powder, which can be made into tea or used in gelatin capsules.

AUTUMN CROCUS. *Colchicum autumnale.* This plant is mentioned because it should never be taken by herbal medicine enthusiasts in its raw form. Any part of the plant may cause death. The gout medicine colchicine is still extracted from the flowers by pharmaceutical firms because it cannot be economically synthesized.

BAEL. *Aegle marmelos.* Called Indian bael or Bengal quince, this traditional medicine came with immigrants from India and Ceylon. The fruit has a hard shell, but is segmented like an orange and the seeds are surrounded by a gummy flesh. The seeds can easily be grown in warmer parts of the United States and when discarded often come up as volunteers. It is used as a calmative for upset stomach and as an astringent, but is almost a specific (a drug or herb used frequently or exclusively for one purpose) for dysentery and diarrhea among East Indian peoples.

BALM. *Melissa officinalis.* Commonly referred to as lemon balm or sweet balm, this herb is often grown for its lemony flavor and fragrance. A member of the mint family, Labiatae, it is effective against stomach upset and is used by herbalists in herbal teas as a carminative, sedative, diaphoretic, and febrifuge. Both the tea and the salve have antibacterial properties; the salve is used in treating surface skin lesions of *Herpes simplex* and other eruptions.

Lemon balm, sometimes called melissa, is also used in treating menstrual cramps, headaches, and nervous stomach. It is said that the ancient Arabs used it to alleviate depression and anxiety. I have used it while cramming for college exams and it helped to relax me. In addition, it is used in some commercial as well as herbal cosmetics and perfumes. The Irish herbalist K'Eogh recommended the leaves, crushed, as a poultice for bee stings.

BALMONY. *Chelone glabra.* Known as turtle head because of the shape of the flowers, balmony was a favorite appetite stimulant among the Native Americans. This bitter herb stimulates digestive action, and is mixed with other herbs, such as lemon balm, so that it is palatable. To make a tea, use one teaspoon of balmony per pint of boiling water and other herbs to taste. Drink about two ounces at a time until normal bowel sounds can be heard or the stomach can be felt moving. This herb tastes much like Angostura bitters to me.

Homeopaths use a tincture of the leaves in water for jaundice and sluggish liver function.

Some say that balmony works as an antidepressant, which may be due to its stimulant qualities. Balmony is collected in wet areas

Liver Tea

1 ounce balmony leaves
1 ounce dried dandelion leaves

Steep the herbs in 1 quart boiling water with a lid on until cool enough to drink. Take 1 to 2 ounces every four hours.

of North America and can be found as a perennial in many gardens, cultivated for its blooms which appear in early fall.

BALSAM FIR. *Abies balsamea.* Other sources may list the scientific name as *Terebinthine canadensis.* At least nine species are found in the wild across Canada and in the United States as far west as Minnesota and south to the Appalachians. Balsam fir makes an excellent Christmas tree, and silviculture (the commercial tree business) has extended its natural range considerably. Native Americans used the gum to heal sores, cuts, and burns, and herbalists make a salve for the same complaints. The resin works so well that it was listed in the *U.S. Pharmacopeia,* the U.S. government's official list of approved medicine. Cherokees and others brewed a tea for chest pains from the inner bark. Needles that turn brown lose their strength, but green needles can be harvested and dried for later use or used fresh to produce a tea for mouth sores and as a laxative.

Balsam needles were thrown on the coals and hot rocks in Indian sweat lodges to relieve congestion of the chest and head, and to stop coughs and colds.

BAMBOO. *Phyllostachys nigra.* This plant was brought to America mainly as an ornamental but now grows in the wild. The leaves can be found in Asian medicine shops as *chu-ju* and are used to treat asthma, coughs, bloody sputum, and fevers due to stress. The sap is called *chu-li* and is used topically for its cooling properties to relieve burns, allay thirst, and stop coughing.

BARBERRY. *Berberis vulgaris.* This bush, which was brought to America from Europe and Britain, is known to most people as a widely naturalized red or green ornamental plant. In the Orient, barberry bushes are grown for their effectiveness as a medicine against bacillary dysentery and diarrhea. The chemical berberine is extracted and has been found to be antibacterial, especially against *Escherichia coli, Streptococcus, Pseudomonas,* and *Salmonella* bacteria.

A tea in the standard proportion of one ounce to one pint of water is used to reduce blood pressure and fight infections in sore throats and is even soaked into poultices or dressings for the treatment of pinkeye. Many herbalists believe that barberry stimulates the immune system and helps to shrink tumors.

Berberine has been included in commercially produced eye drops and in medicines designed to combat diarrhea associated with cholera. The medicinal tea (see recipe) is bitter, but a jelly can be made from the fruits.

Barberry Tea

½ teaspoon powdered root bark
1 cup water
honey to taste

Boil the root powder 15 to 30 minutes. Add honey to alleviate bitterness.

BARLEY. *Hordeum vulgare distochon.* Barley or pearl barley is most commonly known as either a soup grain or an ingredient in malts for whiskey making. However, it has long been used in folk medicine as a nutrient and treatment for bowel inflammation and sore throats, because of its demulcent properties. In these instances, the water in which the barley has been cooked is drunk as a tea. The cooked seeds are also effective in the treatment of rheumatic and arthritic conditions because the levels of sodium in the seeds help to maintain a high serum calcium level. Barley water is good as a dietary supplement but is especially useful in children and infants with recurrent diarrhea. It is gentle on their systems and helps maintain electrolyte balance. Barley can be purchased in grocery or health food stores, although it's usually more expensive in the latter.

Barley Water

2 ounces pearl barley
1 teaspoon lemon juice
5 pints water
1 tablespoon raisins

Boil barley in one pint water until tender, adding raisins
and lemon juice as the barley cools. Strain. Serve the barley as a grain dish or add to other recipes. Add remaining
four pints of water to barley water and simmer down to
two pints. Cool.

Barley water may be soaked into a poultice or cotton and placed
over the eyes while resting to relieve eye strain and dryness. This in
turn may relieve headaches.

BASIL. *Ocimum basilicum.* Basil is another herb that has been used for
centuries as a medicine and as a seasoning. Irish immigrants believed that basil invigorates the nerves. Its aromatic quality does
sharpen the sensations of smell. Bruise basil leaves in vinegar and
hold under the nose to treat fainting. It has long been considered an
aphrodisiac in many cultures.

BAYBERRY. *Myrica cerifera.* The wax found on bayberries has been
harvested for making aromatic candles for centuries. It is used med-
ically as a stimulant, diaphoretic, and cough remedy. A tea is made
from the leaves for cough and sore throat associated with colds.
Powdered bark is added to poultices for sores and ulcers or taken
internally for stomach ulcers. Some Indians chewed the bark and
twigs for relief of fevers while others made a leaf tea for a vermifuge and anesthetic to relieve pain. The Lumbees, a Native

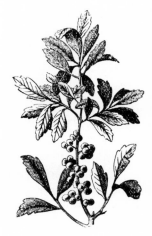

Bayberry

American tribe who lived in the area that is now North and South Carolina, chewed the freshly harvested roots for stomach ulcers, and made a bathing wash from the leaves to treat itching and inflammation on the skin.

A tea was found helpful in treating cankers in the mouth as well as bleeding and irritated gums and as a gargle for sore throats. Bayberry's medicinal taste is pleasant.

Bayberry Tea

1 ounce powdered bark
1 pint water

Simmer bark in water for 20 to 30 minutes. Drink while still warm, about one or two cupfuls total per day.

BEE BALM. *See* Oswego tea.

BEECH. *Fagus grandifolia.* The beech is one of the stateliest trees in the forests of the eastern and central United States. It is possibly the only large tree with smooth, gray bark, making it easy to recognize. The beech is the tree on which Daniel Boone carved the message that he had "killed a bar." (A replica of that tree trunk is on display in the museum at Grandfather Mountain in Linville, North Carolina.) Beech nuts, the tree's triangular seeds, can be eaten raw, and are very effective as a caffeineless substitute for coffee when roasted, ground, and brewed. Beechnut coffee is regularly drunk in some parts of Appalachia.

The bark or leaves, with their astringent effect, can be prepared as a decoction for rinsing poison oak and ivy sores or burns. This astringency is present in a tea for increasing the appetite, for use as a tonic, and for treatment of diarrhea. The tea tends to soothe the stomach as well. Make a tea of ¼ teaspoon ground bark or one teaspoon of crushed leaves and one cup boiling water and take three or four times a day.

Russian immigrants recognized this tree from their own forests back in Russia, where its sap is distilled into a tar or creosote and used for colds, or catarrh as it was known then. They called it *buk.*

BELLADONNA. *Atropa belladonna.* This plant is called deadly nightshade for a good reason and is only mentioned as one to absolutely avoid for internal medications. *All* parts of the plant can be deadly. Today, it is most commonly used by eye doctors in a solution for dilating the pupils. I have had my own eyes dilated with it at the V.A. hospital. Belladonna can be translated from the Italian as "pretty lady," so named because women in that country at one time used it to widen their pupils, to give them that "bedroom look." Atropine, derived from this plant, is used by the military as an antidote to nerve gas.

The herbalist can use belladonna leaves to make a salve or ointment, which is used to treat the pain of gout and arthritis. Some commercial antispasmodics and anticonvulsants are made from belladonna and its synthetic derivatives.

BILBERRY. *Vaccinium myrtillus.* Also known both as huckleberry and as whortleberry, the bilberry is native to northern North America as well as northern Europe, including Britain. Historically, bilberry tea has been drunk for ophthalmological conditions including myopia, night blindness, and, more recently, eye strain. My wife drinks it to relieve the eye strain that comes with being in front of a computer screen all day, a hazard of many modern jobs. It has also been used to treat varicose veins, bleeding gums, hemorrhages, and other circulatory system–related disorders, including phlebitis. Chemicals called anthocyanosides allow increased synthesis of collagen and mucopolysaccharides, which help to stabilize arterial walls. Although sold as a tea in health food stores, the therapeutic proportion is the stronger one ounce of herb to one pint of water. The fresh fruits are used to produce the standardized extract and are mostly wildcrafted, or harvested in the wild.

BIRCH. *Betula* species. Birch bark is so aromatic, with its wintergreen scent, that it was almost eradicated from the Appalachian mountains in the nineteenth century, as Native Americans, herbalists, and commercial pharmaceutical companies all harvested the leaves and twigs to make wintergreen oil. Containing methyl salicylate, it was effective in ointments and salves for sore muscles and sprains. In folk medicine, the oil was extracted from the leaves by boiling them in water or alcohol and was used internally for rheumatism. Birch leaves and / or bark are made into a tea by steeping one teaspoon of the herb in one cup of water for 15 minutes, covered. Charcoal made from birch wood is used as a remedy for absorbing poison from the stomach and digestive tract. The sap is used to make birch beer—both alcoholic and nonalcoholic—and can be reduced by boiling to make syrup.

BLACKBERRY. *Rubus villosus* and many other *Rubus* species. One of my early claims to fame came when the Rodale Institute called to ask me what I knew about herbal and natural remedies for diarrhea. My contribution in their *Doctor's Book of Home Remedies* under the category "Traveler's Diarrhea," and one of my main remedies, is blackberry tea. Almost all parts of this wide-ranging vine, which the English call brambleberry, are useful. Berries, leaves, roots, and root bark are all effectively brewed into a tea (together or separately) for treating diarrhea in a gentle way, unlike some antidiarrheals that cause cramping and pain. Some people like to soak blackberries in vodka or wine to make a cordial that is used to treat diarrhea.

Blackberry roots, leaves, or fruits can be soaked in either hot wine or hot water and gargled for sore throat or rinsed in the mouth for mouth sores or blisters. Blackberry tea is also taken to reduce fevers and to combat excessive menstrual flow.

BLACK COHOSH. *Cimicifuga racemosa.* The Latin name *cimicifuga* translates as "bug repellant" and reflects the plant's use in warding off insects. The plant is an American native, the word "cohosh" coming from an Algonquian word meaning "rough"; it refers to the plant's knobby root, which is used in brewing a tea to counteract menstrual cramps and pains of childbirth. Early settlers called this plant squaw root because it was such a standard Indian remedy for these complaints. This member of the buttercup, or ranunculus, family has been used as a sedative, a relaxant, and an antispasmodic to eliminate stomach spasms. Medical research has shown this herb to be effective for treating PMS and high blood pressure, but it should be used very carefully because of its sedative effect on the central nervous system.

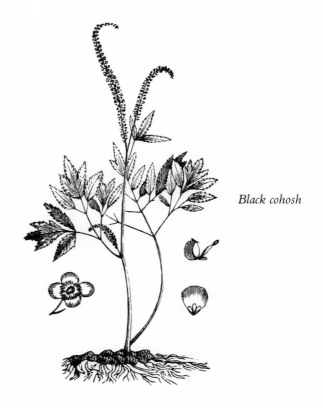

Black cohosh

BLACK WALNUT. *Juglans nigra.* One of the six walnut species native to North America, black walnut is very rich in manganese, important in maintaining the health of the brain, nerves, and cartilaginous tissue. It is best known as a hardwood used in making cabinets, furniture, and gun stocks. Among herbalists, black walnut is most commonly used as a vermifuge, as an elixir or spirit extract to calm hysteria, and especially for its value as an antifungal. My family has had considerable experience with black walnut hulls used as an antifungal. A friend gave my daughter a kitten that had been born and raised under a farmhouse. It was infested with ring-worm sores and spores and we all soon developed this fungal infection. (Ringworm is not a worm at all, but a fungus that forms round patterns on the skin.) I boiled a quantity of walnut hulls—the aromatic green part that surrounds the actual nut—and added this brown fluid to a bathtub full of water. We all soaked in it and the problem was quickly eliminated.

Be aware that walnut hulls also produce a strong dye, which is used to dye horse harnesses, baskets, and other craft items. While in California, I was approached by a woman who was suffering from athlete's foot, another fungal infection. I told her to boil walnut hulls and soak her feet. She boiled the hulls in the morning, allowed them to steep all day, and then reboiled them in the evening. She then soaked her lower legs for several hours while watching television. She called and cursed me because her legs had turned black to just below her knees. They stayed that way for over a week.

If the hulls are not available, use fresh or dried leaves to make a tea for intestinal parasites and diarrhea or a wash for external sores and fungal problems. Black walnut leaves and hulls can be added to shampoos to keep dark hair dark and prevent some scalp diseases. The astringency of black walnuts may require the use of some skin softener such as aloe after use if the skin appears very dry.

BLADDERWRACK. *Fucus vesiculosus.* This seaweed, easily recognized by the air pockets, or bladders, embedded throughout its fronds, is found on both coasts of North America as well as Europe's Atlantic coast. A jellylike substance fills the bladders. The entire plant can be eaten fresh or dried as a treatment for disorders that involve a deficiency of iodine. Alcohol extracts the healing properties for use on external sores, rheumatism, and lumbago, as well as sprains. Bladderwrack pills are available at health food stores, but it can be harvested to use fresh or dried for later. When made into a syrup, the dried leaves alleviate sore throat pain. An ointment made with the mucilage eases dried, cracked skin and promotes healing.

BLESSED THISTLE. *Cnicus benedictus.* This well-known herb, so named because it was grown by monks in Europe, is now naturalized in much of the United States. Herbalists today make a blessed thistle tea for treating liver ailments, fever due to respiratory ailments, febrile conditions, cancer, and heart problems—a use that was mentioned in Shakespeare's writings. It is also used as a contraceptive tea, and can be found in commercial contraceptive preparations.

BLOODROOT. *Sanguinaria canadensis.* Known to American Indians as *puccoon*, this member of the poppy family was given its name because the root "bleeds" when cut or broken. The root is the most commonly used part, but the whole herb contains medicinal properties and has been used in herbal and commercial preparations for centuries. Bloodroot was used in the treatment of cancers, joint swelling, and sore throats, but the FDA calls it unsafe because it is a central nervous system depressant, and great care should be taken in its use. The dried root is very caustic and has been used for removing nose polyps, skin cancers, and warts. Modern medical research has verified its properties as an escharotic and supports its use to remove warts and polyps. Bloodroot was used in topical ointments in the 1800s for treatment of breast tumors. Solutions made from the root were used as a dental analgesic and today are used in commercial preparations and toothpastes for their antiplaque properties. Look for bloodroot in medicines listed as sanguinaria (this is its former name, which also refers to bleeding). In many areas, it is protected as a wildflower.

BLUE COHOSH. *Caulophyllum thalictroides.* Like black cohosh, this is a native plant. Blue cohosh is in a different botanical family from black, but it, too, is called cohosh because of its Native American name. Most specifically blue cohosh was given to women in childbirth. Like black cohosh, it is also known as squaw root, although blue cohosh is in the barberry family. It may also be referred to as yellow ginseng or blue ginseng. Popular in African-American folk medicine as a parturifacient, emmenagogue, and antispasmodic, blue cohosh is used in many herb combinations associated with childbirth. The seeds are poisonous, but the roots are used in powder form to make a tea that is drunk for about two weeks before the due date.

In scientific studies performed in India, rats given a low dose of blue cohosh were seen to exhibit uterine changes that inhibited ovulation. This might be seen to support the herb's use by some Native Americans as a contraceptive.

As a postpartum treatment in a one-to-one combination with pennyroyal, the resultant tea is said to normalize the menstrual cycle.

BONESET. *Eupatorium perfoliatum.* Other plants may be known as boneset—comfrey, for example. This plant is called boneset because it was used to treat breakbone fever, also known as dengue and characterized by acute joint pain. It is used in many cases for its ability to break fevers and its anti-inflammatory properties. A tea is made using two teaspoons to two tablespoons—about one ounce— of the crushed herb, leaves, and flowers, to a pint of water. It is thought to stimulate the immune system and has been used historically to treat colds, influenza, arthritis, and even constipation.

The dried herb is used in making teas. The fresh herb, however, should be avoided because it may cause nausea and vomiting, although this property is sometimes intentionally used to eject poisons from the stomach.

BORAGE. *Borago officinalis.* If borage were an illegal drug it would be known as an "upper," for ever since the time of Pliny, the Roman naturalist, it has been used for lifting the spirits. This European import came with colonists, who had it in their cooking gardens, and is popular today for its cucumberlike flavor when a tea is made from the leaves and flowers. Its recognized medical uses include serving as a demulcent for sore throats and other irritated membranes, as an antipyretic to reduce fevers, and as a poultice. Recent trends tend to warn against borage's use as an internal medicine because it can overstimulate the central nervous system and may cause miscarriage. It is frequently recommended in salves for sores and burns.

BOUNCING BET. *Saponaria officinalis.* Taken internally, this plant should be used only as an emetic and even then with great care. The colonists brought this herb from England and used it as a diuretic. Its common name, soapwort, indicates its use in making a lather for washing the hands or clothes. The Pennsylvania Dutch used and continue to use it to give a foamy head to beer. Externally the crushed herb leaves are applied fresh or in ointments to sores, psoriasis, and acne and are used as a rinse for poison ivy. It thoroughly cleanses the skin with chemicals known as saponins, natural cleaning agents, which make a rich lather when it is used as a liquid soap. Bouncing Bet is widespread in the wild and is grown in many gardens.

BROCCOLI. *Brassica oleracea* var. *italica* [*botrytis cymosa*]. In the country doctor's day, broccoli was eaten raw for preventing stomach and colon cancers, and as a source of provitamin A, vitamin C, and vitamin K. Research has verified the effectiveness of broccoli and other cruciferous vegetables in fighting and preventing various cancers. Researchers at Johns Hopkins University have identified one of these cancer-fighting chemicals as isothiocyanate sulfopharophane. Now, former president George Bush and others who refuse to eat broccoli can obtain its health benefits in commercially produced BCE, or broccoli cruciferous extract.

BROOM. *Cytisus scoparius.* Also known as Scotch broom, this plant, which came from the northern British Isles, has naturalized itself in Africa, North America, and Asia. Once recommended as a cathartic and diuretic, it is considered dangerous by the FDA. I would recommend its use only as a last-ditch attempt to remove dangerous toxins from the bowels. It can stimulate labor in pregnant women and is unpredictable.

BUCKHORN. *See* Plaintain herb.

BURDOCK. *Arctium lappa.* Found throughout Europe and North America as a wild plant, burdock is grown in Asian cultures as a food and called *gobo*. The fresh first-year roots are used as a food rich in fiber and starch. The dried roots are used in herbal medicine as diuretics, diaphoretics, and as alteratives to restore health. As a decoction it is said to be a blood purifier. Its leaves are used in poultices for treatment of sores and skin eruptions.

BUTCHER'S BROOM. *Ruscus aculeatus.* This evergreen shrub is a member of the lily family and was originally found in the Mediterranean area. It is called Butcher's broom because Greek butchers used the stiff twigs to sweep their work areas. It was brought to America by Greek immigrants; the Greeks have used the rhizome for centuries to make a tea that is taken internally for retinal hemorrhaging, and for cramps and other menstrual problems. It can also be made into a salve that is used externally for hemorrhoids, fissures, and varicose veins. Many European women who work as bakers and in other jobs where they must stand all day traditionally have used this salve to reduce varicose veins and prevent and reduce edema of the lower extremities. Occasionally, people have had some allergic reactions, such as nausea or gastritis.

CACAO. *Theobroma cacao.* The Aztecs were using the products of the cacao plant when it was "discovered" by the Spanish conquistador Hernando Cortez and taken back to Spain. From there it went to England and then came back to this country in the 1600s. Cocoa is made from the dried and ground cacao beans and makes an effective pick-me-up because it is a gentle stimulant; since it contains only about ⅙ the caffeine of coffee we don't experience the jitters and irritability that coffee may bring nor the headaches when we quit drinking it for an extended period of time. The chemical theobromine in cocoa relaxes the smooth muscle that lines the digestive tract, aiding digestion and making it effective against cramps. Most people today get their cacao in the form of chocolate candy, a fairly recent use for this native medication for asthma. The theobromine and caffeine help to relax the bronchial passages and also help in flu and cold symptoms. Serve hot cocoa with your chicken soup in cold season!

CALAMUS. *Acorus calamus.* Also called sweet flag, this wetland plant is known to us from traditional Native American use and from biblical passages as an anointing herb. It is found in the Middle East, China, and North America.

The aromatic rhizome is used both to fight flatulence and as a carminative. It is known to treat dyspepsia and to have expectorant activity as well. The roots were chewed by the Cherokees, Lumbees, and Saponis as a stimulant and believed by some to be an aphrodisiac. It has also been used in the past by physicians to treat stomach cramps and to provide a tonic stimulant.

Calamus can easily be confused with wild blue iris, which has similar leaves and grows in the same habitats. Calamus can be distinguished by its small brown flower cones, which jut from the leaves; iris has the fleur-de-lis–shaped flowers that often are used as a symbol on crests. Also, calamus has a distinct aroma and iris is scentless. Calamus has been cooked down to sugar syrup and made into a candy. The FDA reported that calamus bought on the open market should be considered unsafe because rhizomes of Asian origin have been shown to cause cancer in rats.

CALENDULA. *See* Marigold.

CAMPHOR. *Cinnamomum camphora.* Camphor is a gum or distillate from the bark of the camphor tree, which grows in China and Japan. Distilled oil of camphor was a stock item for the country doctor, and is still used today in many medications for relief of pain, cold sores, and stiff muscles. Small doses have been used to relieve diarrhea, but it is recommended for external use only.

CARAWAY. *Carum carvi.* Most people know caraway as the seeds on their rye bread or the seasoning in sauerkraut, but this member of the parsley family has been used for thousands of years as a digestive aid and to calm the stomach and expel gas. Some women have used a tea of caraway seeds to alleviate cramping and uterine contractions during menstruation and after childbirth. To make a tea, crush three teaspoons of seeds and steep them in boiling water. You might want to put a lid on the pot because covered teas retain their volatile oils better than uncovered ones. Caraway is easy to grow from seeds in a garden, where it also attracts black swallowtail butterflies, as do other members of the parsley family. It likes full sun and rich soil that drains quickly after a rain. You can grow it in pots year-round or, in mild climates, with successive plantings.

CARDAMOM. *Elettaria cardamomum.* The seeds of this readily available kitchen spice are ground and made into a tea that calms the stomach and serves well as a carminative. Cardamom comes from the Malabar coast of India as well as other places and was brought here in the course of trade with the British Empire, like the majority of nonnative commercial spices. It has long been valued for its antispasmodic action when used as a spice or taken as a tea.

CARDINAL FLOWER. *Lobelia cardinalis.* This member of the lobelia family is characterized by bright red flowers and is protected in some states. It blooms along muddy creek banks and in other wet spots. Cherokees used it as a remedy for syphilis, but it is best known as Indian tobacco and is used to help wean people from nicotine (although no one is sure exactly how it works). It is rarely used today except for such purposes.

CASCARA SAGRADA. *Rhamnus purshiana.* Also known as buckthorn, the dried bark of this plant of the Pacific Northwest is used to make laxatives, cathartics, purgatives, and liver tonics, and to help restore tone to the liver. The bark, identified by the Spanish translation of its name as "sacred bark," is stripped from the plants in spring, dried, and pulverized. It can be purchased and taken as powder in capsules, or in commercial preparations as an elixir. Elixir of cascara sagrada is one of the "drugs" given in military hospitals for constipation. It should not be taken by persons with irritable bowel syndrome. In standardized preparations, a dose of 50 to 100 milligrams of 25 percent HAD (hydroxy anthracene derivate) is used for constipation, producing a stool in about six hours or so under normal circumstances. A stronger dose is used as a cathartic.

Laxatives should only be used occasionally to relieve constipation, after fiber in the diet, hydration, and exercise have failed to produce results. One should try a gentler bulk-forming laxative such as psyllium first. Also, do not give cascara sagrada to children under two years of age, to ulcer patients, or to pregnant women.

CATNIP. *Nepeta cataria.* Amazingly, this member of the mint family acts as a stimulant on felines and serves as a sedative and tranquilizer for humans. The Chinese and Europeans have used it for at least 2,000 years, so it is well tested and documented. It is also used as an emmenagogue and the leaves can be chewed to relieve toothache. The chemicals in catnip that have been identified as nepetalactone isomers are similar to those found in valerian, the natural source for Valium. The colonists brought catnip here and now it grows wild virtually everywhere, but you still may want to grow your own, bearing in mind that you will often find cats wallowing in it.

CAYENNE. *Capsicum annuum, C. frutescens,* and *C. minimum.* It is said that the best cayenne, also called capsicum, comes from Zanzibar, but an excellent variety also comes from Louisiana—the world-famous cayenne pepper grown especially for and by the McIlhenny family and used in the production of Tabasco sauce. Cayenne is listed as an ingredient in many medicines, as is the chemical capsaicin, which is obtained from it. Cayenne has long been used by herbalists to make a salve to relieve the pain of swollen joints and arthritis, and many commercial products now boast capsaicin as an ingredient, even the main ingredient. Some even use it in the name of their medication. Cayenne is high in vitamin C, turns on the body's thermostat, induces sweating, increases coronary output, and promotes digestion. A wide variety of commercial over-the-counter medicines take advantage of cayenne's ability to increase blood flow and cardiac output.

One male sex stimulant advertised as improving potency and sexual vigor was bought by a coworker of mine—at a cost of $1 a capsule. After the purchase, the curious patron asked if it was safe and if it would work. The only ingredient was ground cayenne—red pepper. Yes, it does help, because men depend on good blood flow to be able to achieve erection, but if purchased as a spice $1 would buy a lot more cayenne! Arthritis and herpes medicines typically use capsaicin as the only healing ingredient, at a strength of .025 percent, or one fourth of 1 percent, which at around $40 a tube makes it a very expensive pinch of red pepper! Made into a tea, cayenne is excellent for increasing body warmth.

Winter-Warmer Cayenne Tea

¼ teaspoon ginseng concentrate
½ teaspoon ground cayenne pepper
1 teaspoon honey
1 cup water
½ teaspoon ground fresh ginger

Pour boiling water over other ingredients and let steep, covered, for 10 minutes. Stir well and drink all at once. Be ready to sweat!

Cayenne has a multitude of uses. During the Civil War and since, it has been used in the relief of delirium tremens in alcoholics and to combat constipation, cough, nausea, joint pain, and shingles. Hodgkin's disease sufferers have been relieved of their postherpetic neuralgia pain with an application of cayenne salve.

Homemade Cayenne Liniment

1 cup warm olive oil
½ teaspoon ground cayenne

Mix and allow to sit for several days if possible so that the capsaicin will be distributed throughout the oil. Other vegetable oils may be used.

By carefully reducing the strength of capsaicin so that it does not burn sensitive skin, you can use it to treat cluster headaches by rubbing a little just inside the nostrils and on the bridge of the nose.

CASTOR OIL. *Ricinus communis.* Castor oil was a standby of the country doctor and my mother as a spring tonic and cleanser. Today, it is commonly sold as a laxative in stores. However, since there are so many safer laxatives available, castor oil should be used only externally or in hospitals where it is used to clean out the bowel effectively before radiological examination. Castor oil comes from the cold pressing of castor beans after the seed skin is removed, a process that should not be attempted by the home or amateur herbalist. An extremely toxic poison called ricin is extracted from the seed skins and is so dangerous that possession of this chemical is a violation of the 1989 Biological Weapons Antiterrorism Act and conviction can lead to life imprisonment! Castor oil is effective in external application as an emollient; it is used in racing car engines to reduce friction!

CELERY SEED. *Apium graveolens.* Celery seed has been shown to be effective in lowering blood sugar, making it effective in the management of diabetes. A tea made of two to three teaspoons of bruised seeds per cup of boiling water, taken up to three times a day, makes an excellent diuretic and also helps to lower blood pressure. This tea has also been used to promote menstruation. Some studies on rodents have shown the tea to have an antiepileptic action. Celery seed's reputation as an aphrodisiac is not proven.

CHAMOMILE. Some confusion exists around chamomile because there are at least two distinct varieties: German chamomile is *Matricaria chamomilla*; and Roman chamomile is *Anthemis nobilis*—two separate species with similar actions and uses. Though standardized products are available, many people prefer to grow their own chamomile—but wild plants are believed to be stronger than culti-

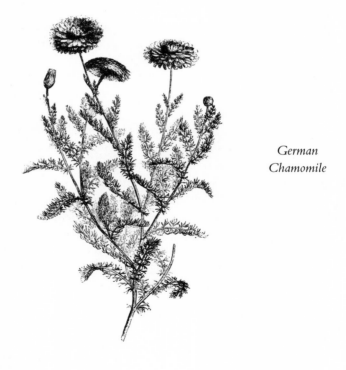

German Chamomile

vated ones. The flower, the most-used part, is harvested when fully open and is dried for later use (the leaves are sometimes used as well).

Historically, chamomile has been used as a painkiller, muscle relaxant, antiseptic, tonic, sedative, and calmative. The Germans call it *alles zutraut*, meaning "capable of anything," because of its many uses. Perhaps known best for its soothing effect on the nerves, chamomile tea is used to relax, reduce anxiety and stress, and promote sleep. It produces a safe state of gentle relaxation without inhibiting awareness or inducing a state of grogginess and reduced reaction time. The tea can also be used as a wash or rinse to ward off insects. It is made with one or two tablespoons of flowers per cup of water. The strained tea can be put in a baby's bottle to prevent stomachaches in small children. Chamomile tea can also be made into a nice jelly by substituting the tea for apple juice or other juice and adding pectin as called for.

Chamomile is gaining popularity with those who wish to give up nicotine and tobacco. The flowers, eaten straight or made into cookies and consumed when the urge for tobacco strikes, are said to be an effective deterrent. Some persons clear their congested nasal passages using inhalation therapy and chamomile flowers. Others use the flowers in a cloth bag suspended in running bath water for its relaxing effect and to make sleep easier.

CHASTE TREE, CHASTE BERRY. *Vitex agnus-castus.* The dried fruits of this European tree have long been used to repress sexual desire, thus the common name. It is also known as monk's pepper. Historically it has been used in the treatment of dysmenorrhea, amenorrhea, menopause symptoms, and premenstrual tension, as well as to relieve mood swings and tension due to nerves and insomnia. Tablets are available and are said to be equally effective. The wild berries are harvested mainly in Israel, as they have been for ages. It is rumored that the berries were secretly added to the food of Jewish teenagers to distract their interest in the opposite sex.

CHICKWEED. *Stellaria* species. This common weed is used in weight-loss diets and products under the name stellaria, which means "starlike" and refers to the flowers. Chickweed is high in vitamin C and may be eaten raw or added to salads, soups, and stir-fry dishes. Chickweed ointment is used to treat boils, ulcers, bedsores, and eczema.

CHINESE ANGELICA. *See* Dong quai.

CINNAMON. *Cinnamomum verum.* Cinnamon oil and cinnamon sticks have long been used to treat stomach upset and as a carminative. In Mexico it is widely believed that burning cinnamon sticks as incense will sexually stimulate women. Cinnamon is mentioned on several occasions in the Bible and in the classic herbals. Eugenol, an oil also found in cloves, is effective in treating toothache, but must be diluted to protect nerves in the tooth.

CLEAVERS. *Galium aparine.* This common wild plant is also known as bed straw because it was actually used as such, as goose grass because it is a favorite food of geese, and as madder because it is in the madder family, though other plants share this name. Cleavers, which produces a red dye, is effective for vitamin C deficiency. Also, its tiny seeds can be roasted and brewed into a caffeine-free coffee substitute. Salves made with cleavers have been used to treat psoriasis.

CLOVES. *Sysigum aromaticum.* The name "cloves" comes from the Greek word meaning "nail" and refers to the shape of the clove buds, which resemble the nails used to hold Jesus on the cross. The cloves that most of us are familiar with are roasted flower buds and are the source of eugenol, used in home and commercial toothache remedies. Bruised cloves can be rolled in the mouth for toothache relief but should not be chewed, as the oil can damage the nerves

the same way to stimulate appetite, lower blood-sugar levels, and boost sluggish immune systems. Devil's claw gets its name from the shape of its fruits, which resemble a great claw. It is now found in health food stores as a standardized extract. It should be avoided during pregnancy as it has been shown to stimulate the uterine muscle and could cause abortion, miscarriage, or a premature birth. The British Herbal Pharmacopoea recognizes devil's claw for treating dyspepsia and rheumatism and for its sedative qualities.

DEVIL'S CLUB. *Olopanax horridus.* This plant is native to the Pacific Northwest, Canada, and Alaska; in the language of native Alaskans, it's known as *cukilanarpak,* which means "large plant with needles." Devil's club grows in moist ravines and may reach a height of 15 feet or more. Its large stem is thickly studded with thorny growths. The prickly outer bark is used to make decoctions and poultices, and the inner bark, or cambium, is chewed in the traditional treatment of body pain, wounds, and arthritis, or to produce an emetic or purgative effect. Frontier doctors and native healers use this plant in the treatment of diabetes due to its hypoglycemic actions.

DEVIL'S DUNG. *Ferula assafoetida.* Sometimes called asafetida, this herb has a characteristic odor and a taste that's stronger than that of onions. It is indigenous to Iran and Afghanistan but has long been popular among African Americans for the treatment of abdominal tumors, asthma, convulsions, insanity, and cancer. The resin is also used as an expectorant and carminative. Its main use today is as a preservative in candy and perfume. The resin is available in pharmacies and health food and ethnic stores. It may be found growing in some parts of this country where it has been introduced.

DILL. *Anthemum graveolens.* This familiar herb is used in cooking fish and potato dishes, and in making candies and pickles. Among herbalists, the seeds are regarded as infection fighters and digestive aids when made into a tea or consumed whole (raw or cooked).

Dill seeds can also be chewed to freshen the breath. The old granny saying "If a kid has colic, let him suck a pickle" refers to the gas-dispelling qualities of dill. Dill helps relax the smooth muscles of the digestive tract. Research has shown that dill oil inhibits the growth of some bacteria. Dill tea is believed to reduce blood pressure by stimulating respiration, slowing the heart rate, and opening blood vessels.

DODDER. *Cuscuta epithymum.* Dodder, or love weed, has long been used in tea form to treat kidney infections and ailments. It is a leafless parasitic vine that is related to the morning glory and twines over fields across this country. The English herbalist Nicholas Culpeper believed it was effective against melancholia or depression.

DOGWOOD. *Cornus florida.* The state tree of Virginia and state flower of North Carolina and other states was well known to the country doctor as the ague tree. The dried bark of the dogwood was made into a decoction to treat joint pain and fevers. During the Civil War, the bark was boiled and used as a substitute for quinine. The fresh bark is a strong, almost harsh, laxative. The dogwood is reported to be the tree that Jesus was crucified on, and legend has it that this is what caused the tree to be reduced to its present wizened shape. In museums, huge old logs of dogwood attest to its former grandeur and support the legend. The Latin name means "flowered hardwood." The dense wood is used in making golf club heads.

DONG QUAI. *Angelica sinensis.* Chinese angelica is available in standardized form and is taken in doses of 200 milligrams three times a day for all sorts of female problems. In China it's considered the most important female tonic and is used to treat menopausal symptoms, PMS, and uterine cramping. Chills of the feet and hands, anemia, and general tiredness have also responded well to dong quai. The dried root of this herb is the part used and it can be grown or purchased and made into a decoction. In commercial production, the roots of three-year-old plants are harvested and the chemical ligustilide and other active substances are distilled using a traditional water-alcohol extraction method.

DYER'S WEED. *Genista tinctoria.* Also called dyer's broom, this European native is cultivated elsewhere and may be encountered here. Herbalists have grown it for its yellow dye, but they also make a tea from the leaves and sticks as a diuretic, emetic, and cathartic. It has been used in the treatment of gout and arthritis.

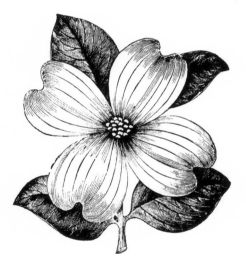

Dogwood blossom

ECHINACEA. *Echinacea purpurea, E. pallida,* and *E. angustifolia.* This is the family of plants, known as coneflowers, that has received so much attention recently from herbal-medicine practitioners and pharmaceutical researchers. The root is the part of the plant that is harvested and used by people around the world for the treatment of immune system disorders and as an antibiotic. Plains Indians used the root to make a wash for skin disorders, a tea to treat colds and fevers, and poultices for wounds, insect bites and stings, and snakebites. They also made an echinacea mouthwash to treat sore teeth and gums, pyorrhea, and gingivitis. Its anti-inflammatory qualities have led German herbalists to use echinacea in a tincture to treat arthritis.

Echinacea Decoction

1 tablespoon ground echinacea root
½ pint water

Bring to a boil and simmer for 15 minutes. The decoction can be sweetened to taste if preferred. Drink one cup three times a day. Commercial preparations are also available with their own instructions.

Initially, echinacea will taste sweet, but then it turns bitter. Some people have reported a tingling of the tongue and mouth when taking echinacea, but there is no known toxicity.

Echinacea, a perennial that readily produces "volunteers," is easily grown in the home flower garden. The roots are ready for harvesting when the plant is about four years old.

Historically, this herb has also been used to treat tonsillitis and sore throat, to relieve allergic symptoms, and to prevent or relieve water retention. Currently, echinacea is being investigated for its antitumor and anticancer effectiveness and its ability to boost the immune system. A standard product is readily available as an extract or root powder.

Echinacea has also been shown to have antiviral capabilities as well as the ability to kill fungi and bacteria. A wash of echinacea tea is useful in treating yeast infections and is effective in counteracting the effects of radiation therapy. Echinacea tea has also been used in the treatment of meningitis, asthma, and tuberculosis. Echinacea will become the next "wonder drug" if pharmaceutical firms can get a patent on it.

ELDER. *Sambucus nigra, S. canadensis.* Several varieties of elderberry are found in the United States. (In the West, a red-fruited variety is considered unsafe to eat.) The flower, bark, leaf, and fruit of elderberry are used in various medications. A soothing and effective wash for hemorrhoids is made by combining equal amounts of elder and honeysuckle flowers and steeping them in boiled water for up to half an hour. They are then applied as a compress or poultice. Elderberry root is a very powerful purgative and should only be used with care and under supervision.

In England, it is believed that witches are associated with elder shrubs and hide in them. In Mexico, where the elder is known as *saúco*, the flowers are boiled and the steam inhaled to cleanse the skin of impurities. In other places, the flowers are mixed into salves or oil and applied to the skin to aid in the removal of freckles.

The bark can be made into a diuretic and laxative tea, which is used to relieve fluid retention. The crushed fresh leaves are also mixed with olive oil and applied topically to reduce hemorrhoids. It is generally considered unwise to consume the leaves and other green parts. Eat only the ripe berries, which are rather bland when raw, but become sweet with cooking. A jelly made from the berries helps relieve constipation in children.

Elder grows wild throughout America in moist places and in the British Isles and Europe as well.

ELECAMPANE. *Inula helenium.* Also known as horseheal and wild sunflower, this large member of the composite family is native to Europe and Asia, but has naturalized in America. It is found over most of the East from Quebec to Minnesota and south to North Carolina and Missouri. This perennial produces yellow flowers, but the large, gray root is the part used by herbalists. At one time, elecampane was listed in the *U.S. Pharmacopeia* as a treatment for respiratory diseases. In the 1800s the roots were boiled in sugar syrup to make throat lozenges. Today, it is more commonly known for its use in treating skin conditions on horse and sheep, though humans use it, too. For treating coughs and bronchitis, as well as nausea and diarrhea, you can use two to four grams of the powdered root and make a tea or capsule.

ELM. *Ulmus carpinifolia.* These large trees grow in much of the temperate world. In Mexico, the elm is called *olmo.* Herbalists and country doctors have long used the dried bark—after soaking it in cold water overnight and then boiling the bark and water—to relieve edema and peripheral fluid retention. Some people recommend drinking the water left from soaking the bark to clear the complexion. This tea is also soaked into compresses and applied to eruptions of the skin including boils and bedsores to help drain and dry them. The bark decoction contains astringents as well as demulcents so is used to relieve sore throats when gargled and acts as a diuretic when drunk.

EPHEDRA. *Ephedra vulgaris, E. sinica,* and other species. The ephedras have long been used as central nervous system stimulants. The Chinese ephedra known and marketed as *ma huang* has been used for thousands of years as a stimulant for the parasympathetic nervous system and to treat bronchial spasms. Research has shown that it functions as a bronchodilator by stimulating the cardiac muscles and cardiac output, which in turn increases the blood pressure. Ephedra is the source of the alkaloid ephedrine. Laboratory-produced ephedrine and pseudoephedrine has supplanted the use of natural forms in many areas. The natural or synthesized form is used in many cold medicines because it relieves congestion in mucous tissues. A tea can be made of the stem, leaves, and other above-ground parts of this evergreen plant; a standard extract is made by removing the active principle through a water and alcohol solvent method and then evaporating most of the liquid off.

Ephedrine is the synthetic ingredient in cold medicines like Sudafed. Sold commercially as a decongestant, it has been abused by some young people who take the decongestant in large quantities for the rush. As with any drug abuse or misuse, using ephedra to get high can have disastrous—even fatal—effects. Some people have used it in a weight-loss program because it changes the basal metabolic rate, which causes the body to burn more calories while at rest. Ephedra may induce uterine contractions and cause spontaneous abortion. It has been used by some women to promote menstruation.

It has been reported but not proved that some of the wild ephedras of the western United States do not contain the central nervous system stimulants; they are, however, used as beverages and decongestants.

ERGOT. *Claviceps purpurea.* This is rye and corn smut and it is only mentioned because some old herbals suggest its use as a postpartum treatment to control hemorrhaging. Since it is the source of LSD, its value as a vasoconstrictor is far overshadowed by its potential dangers.

EUCALYPTUS. *Eucalyptus* species. A wide variety of eucalyptus trees are now cultivated in North and South America. (These are the huge white trees seen in the television series *Murder She Wrote*, in which they give away the location of the mythical Cabot Cove as southern California and not Maine.) Eucalyptus oil is the aroma we recognize in Vicks VapoRub and other medications used to help open congested bronchial passages.

For treating chest congestion and pain, I have boiled the leaves as part of inhalation therapy; the steam is inhaled with good results. The dried leaves have been smoked in the treatment of asthma. The dried leaves store well and can be crushed to release their oil into salves for making your own "vapor rub" or for adding their pleasant scent and rubefacient qualities to other herbal salves. Olive oil can also be used to extract the decongestant properties from the leaves; rub the therapeutic oil on the chest as needed. The decoction from the leaves is also used to treat dandruff and chapped skin and appears to have some antibiotic properties.

EUPHORBIUM. *Euphorbia resinifera*. Known as crown of thorns, this plant was once recommended as a purgative. Now, however, its effects are believed to be so drastic that it is no longer recommended and is considered one of the poisonous plants of the Christmas season. Because of its toxic properties, it should not be taken in any form.

EVENING PRIMROSE. *Oenothera biennis*. Also called sundrop, the yellow flowers of this garden flower and escapee are a common sight across the country. Much research is now being carried out on the seeds, which are a source of GLA (gamma-linolenic acid), an effective treatment for premenstrual syndrome and high blood pressure. It also works well as an antioxidant. The oil from the seeds is taken in a dose of 250 mg or more daily to promote red blood cell formation. In the country doctor's day, the leaves were made into a poultice to treat skin eruptions and female problems. The effectiveness of the oil in the treatment of schizophrenia, hyperactivity in children, and arthritis is being investigated. It is important not to confuse the evening primrose with the English primrose (*Primula* species), which is poisonous to consume.

Evening primrose oil is sold as a nutritional supplement in more than 30 countries around the world. In the United States the annual production of seeds, which are the size of coarse-ground pepper, surpasses 300 tons.

FENNEL. *Foeniculum vulgare, F. officinalis*, and other species. This member of the parsley family has been used for thousands of years as a medicine. Native to the Mediterranean region, fennel is grown in many parts of the world. In Mexico it is known as *hinojo* and is used as an appetite stimulant and a diuretic. The leaves, seeds, and roots are used in various ways, including being eaten dry, made into teas, and added to food for treatment of flatulence and nausea.

Inhaling the steam of boiling seeds has provided relief for migraines in some people. Some studies suggest a mild estrogenic effect in the seeds, bringing relief of menopause symptoms, promoting menstruation, and acting as a female hormone.

Weak fennel-seed tea is given to small children to relieve colic. The ancient Greeks called fennel *marathon* because it grew wild

Gas Relief Drink

1 cup milk
1 to 2 teaspoons fennel seeds

Heat ingredients almost to a boil and simmer for about 10 minutes. Drink hot to relieve gas and stomach pains. The same mixture is said to promote lactation in nursing mothers.

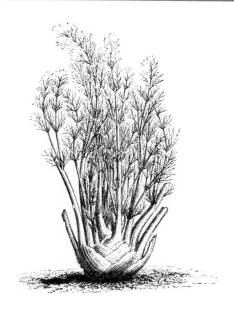

Fennel

around the village of that name. The Puritans of New England called the seeds "meeting seeds" because they were used to suppress the appetite during long church services and because they masked the odor of whiskey on the breath. Fennel came to America with the colonists and is now found as an herb growing in many gardens; it also grows wild in California and other places, where it has escaped and the climate is favorable.

When gathering any herb, positive identification is a key safety factor. It is critical to not confuse wild fennel with its cousin, poison hemlock, a deadly plant, in areas where both grow.

FENUGREEK. *Trigonella foenum-graecum.* This legume, sometimes known as Greek hay, was part of the famous Lydia E. Pinkham's Vegetable Compound (a popular old-time patent medicine) taken for "female weakness." Today, herbalists use fenugreek in poultices for wounds, rashes, boils, and ulcers. Most people come in contact with fenugreek, though, as an ingredient in artificial maple syrup. A decoction of fenugreek helps soothe a sore throat and may bring on menstrual flow. In some parts of the Middle East it is used to treat diabetes. The seeds relieve gas, making it an effective carminative; they also soften the skin when crushed.

FEVERBUSH. *Garrya fremonti.* The leaves of this broad-leaved desert plant, also known as skunkbush or California feverbush, are used as a bitter appetite stimulant and as a ferbrifuge in tea form. This herb has lost a bit of its popularity but is still used by some Native Americans.

FEVERFEW. *Tanacetum parthenium.* This chrysanthemum is a popular treatment for migraine headaches, with relief coming either from chewing the fresh herb or drinking a tea made from the leaves and stems. The fresh leaves when eaten alone have a harsh taste, though some find it tasty. It grows wild in much of Europe and is a popular garden flower and potted plant.

Feverfew is an easily grown perennial herb that reaches a height of three feet and has daisylike flowers with white petals and yellow centers. It can be grown in the garden or in a pot and taken out for sunshine when the weather is good. Extracts have been used to relieve pain of menstruation, arthritis, and asthma. Feverfew is also used as an antipyretic, as a stomachic, to lower blood pressure, and as a digestive aid. Those who suffer from migraine headaches can freeze the leaves of fresh plants for when they are needed.

Today, standardized extracts are made with leaves processed into capsules containing 500 mg of the active ingredient, parthenolide. It may take as long as a month of daily doses before feverfew becomes effective against migraines. Historically, feverfew has also been used to treat depression, encourage restful sleep, and alleviate vertigo. The word "parthenium" comes from a legend that a worker on the Parthenon's roof was saved as he chewed feverfew to prevent dizziness. It has been proved to reduce both histamine production and blood-vessel spasms in migraines.

FIG. *Ficus carica.* Figs come in many varieties and are a fun medicine because they taste good. The country doctor and many people today in the rural South recognize figs as an effective, gentle laxative, as indicated by their small seeds. The fig is actually the flower of the plant; both the male and female flowers are in the "fruit." Figs are mentioned in several places in the Bible as food and medicine. They are emollient and soothing to irritated tissues. In Mexico fig trees are called *higuera* and stewed figs are often used to treat sore throats and coughs. As a skin treatment, the raw fig can be split and applied to boils, tumors, and abscesses. The milky sap is used to treat corns and warts, but care should be taken not to get it in the eyes.

FLAX. *Linum usitatissimum.* This plant is also known as linseed, but herbalists caution against using the flax, or linseed, oil available at hardware stores because of contamination with other seeds and chemicals. Linseed oil has been applied externally to the skin as a demulcent and emollient, and taken internally as a laxative. Some old herbals recommend moistening a flaxseed and placing it against the eyeball with the lid closed to remove foreign matter. The flaxseed swells and produces a mucilage that the irritant sticks to,

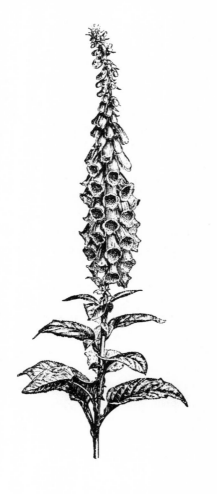

Foxglove

making removal easier. Research suggests that flaxseed oil in the diet is effective in lowering cholesterol and lipids in the bloodstream. The oil is also effective for treating burns and soothing abraded skin.

FOXGLOVE. *Digitalis purpurea.* The foxglove is a potentially fatal plant, especially when mistaken for comfrey, which is similar in appearance if identifying flowers are not present. Foxglove is the only source of digitalis, indispensable in the treatment of many heart conditions; no synthetic drug has been developed as a substitute. Digitalis is still produced from foxgloves. It is used in the professional treatment of certain cardiac conditions, particularly congestive heart failure. Yet it is such a dangerous central nervous system and cardiac depressant in auricular fibrillation (an erratic, rapid heartbeat), that the health hazards easily outweigh any benefits of experiments with the plant. Even the standardized commercial preparation is potentially deadly, so avoid foxglove altogether.

GARLIC. *Allium sativum.* Garlic is my choice for the most popular herb. Known to the Chinese as *hu suan* and to Mexicans as *ajo*, this member of the lily family was used by Cherokee healers as a remedy for asthma, croup, scurvy, and colic. Chinese have used garlic since the sixth century and it is still an official drug in the pharmacopeia of the People's Republic of China. Historically it has been used to fight infections and colds, to prevent gangrene, and as an antibiotic, antifungal, anthelmintic, and antiviral. Recent studies show that it has properties that act against both gram-negative and gram-positive organisms, making it a broad-spectrum antibiotic.

Fresh garlic is always the preferred form of this important medicine. Some believe that as prepared products sit on shelves, they lose potency. Garlic's principle ingredient is alliin, which is high in sulphur. This compound—and garlic itself—promotes wound healing, helps to stop the liver from producing too much cholesterol, and reduces clotting tendencies. Such qualities would have made the country doctor's remedies for ateriosclerosis, high blood pressure, and heart diseases legitimate medical treatments. Today much research is under way to test garlic as an anticancer and antitumor drug and determine its effectiveness in treating pneumonia, whooping cough, diphtheria, and infectious hepatitis. In China, allicin, another garlic extract, is available as an injection to prevent and treat infection.

Country doctors made an effective cough syrup from crushed garlic cloves and brown sugar, a nosebleed remedy by crushing peeled cloves and pressing the paste against the nostril opposite the bleeding one, and an antidiarrhea treatment by pressing a clove into the navel. A peeled garlic clove wrapped in gauze was inserted into the ear to cure earache and was held against an abscess to relieve it and the accompanying toothache.

Before going into the field, I have eaten three or four cloves daily to prevent problems with ticks and mosquitoes. Since it's preventative, it is much safer than the sulphur match-head treatment to rid oneself of attached ticks that is recommended in some military manuals. Furthermore, the garlic provides resistance to infection from cuts, bites, and other skin breaks—not to mention colds and chilblains.

Crushed garlic cloves are added to olive oil or other oils as a treatment for burns and abrasions, insect bites and sores.

Garlic tea is useful for treating stomach ulcers and diarrhea. In Mexico, garlic is crushed and mixed with honey or bread to treat dandruff, wounds, and even scorpion bites. It has also been used historically as a digestive tonic and to prevent and treat gastritis. During World War II European physicians prevented infection and gangrene by applying gauze or another dressing material soaked in garlic juice, which they nicknamed Russian or British penicillin.

Asthma Remedy

1 pint brandy or vodka
4 to 6 cloves garlic

Crush garlic and place in alcohol. Set aside in a dark closet for approximately a week, strain, and take by teaspoonsful to relieve asthmatic coughing or bronchitis.

Indian doctors have used garlic to treat Hansen's disease (leprosy), and European studies have shown that garlic will help the body eliminate lead and other toxic and heavy-metal poisons.

Garlic is a perennial herb and can be grown from cloves or from seed. It is generally planted around Ground Hog Day, or some six weeks before the last frost, in rich, well-drained soil and is harvested in late summer, or when the leaves begin to wither.

GENTIAN. *Gentian campestris* and *G. lutea.* The roots of this European herb were used in the late 1800s to make a medicine called Moxie, which was popular with country doctors for the treatment of various gastrointestinal disorders from poor appetite and gastritis to nausea and heartburn. Today, a decoction of one teaspoon of powdered gentian root in three cups of water is used to treat arthritis, promote menstruation, and stimulate the digestion. Native Americans used *Gentian puberula* (a related, similar herb) to treat back pain, and gentian was listed in the U.S. Pharmacopeia from 1820 to 1955. Today it may be purchased as a tincture and, like other bitter herbs, is promoted as a digestive aid and stimulant.

GINGER. *Zingiber officinale.* Known as Jamaican ginger, African ginger, and cochin ginger, as well as Indian ginger, ginger roots are commonly sold in stores for cooking and these roots can be grown into large plants in the garden. Ginger originated in India, Nigeria, and Israel, but it is now cultivated in many tropical countries. It has a great number of uses, but is best known for treating nausea, vomiting, seasickness and airsickness; for eliminating dizziness and morning sickness in early pregnancy; for increasing and stimulating the appetite; and for fighting colds and cough. Mexican *curanderas* call it *jengibre* and use the leaves as well as the roots to make a tea to relieve general "achy feeling." Ginger water is used to relieve tired or sore feet and slivered or grated ginger is added to bathwater to increase circulation and relieve tired muscles and sore joints.

Ginger is used to raise the body's metabolism and also as a diaphoretic, which increases circulation and eliminates cell toxins and products of infection. I once made a series of training videos for the U.S. Army on edible wild plants of North America. A section shot in

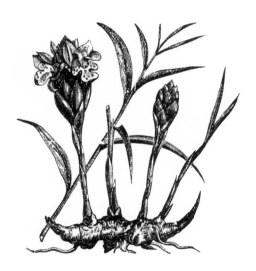

Indian Ginger

June of harvesting cattails in a lake had to be refilmed in January when it was 13 degrees—I had to wear the same rolled-up sleeves as in June. The camera crew took turns warming up in a car with the motor running while I waded into the frozen lake after the cattails. Despite the temperature, sweat poured from my head after I drank a special preparation: using ginseng tea as a base, I added one tablespoon fresh grated ginger and ½ teaspoon cayenne to each cup. After this tea's effect was written up in military papers, it was used to help warm up U.S. Air Force student pilots in unheated training aircraft.

Studies have shown ginger to have a cholesterol-lowering capability and to reduce blood clotting. It is also an antioxidant and an antibiotic as well as an antiflatulant. Its phlegm- and mucus-loosening properties make it an effective expectorant. Some consider ginger an aphrodisiac, but this is likely due to its effect of raising the metabolism and increasing blood flow.

GINGER, WILD. *Asarum canadense.* This native North American plant (see drawing on page 21) is not related to Jamaican ginger; it does, however, have the same characteristic scent and taste in the roots, which are long and slender in contrast to the thickened roots of commercially grown ginger. Wild ginger has heart-shaped evergreen leaves and a brown bell-shaped flower, which is hidden among leaf litter and is pollinated by ants, which are attracted by a rotten-meat scent. Wild ginger is high in aristocholic acid, which in clinical tests in China has been shown to promote healing and prevent infection. It has also been used to reduce the toxic effects of some commercial antibiotics. Native Americans used it as an expectorant, carminative, and stimulant. The Cherokees made a poultice of the leaves and used it to treat wounds and heal bruises.

GINKGO. *Ginkgo biloba.* Commonly known as the maidenhair tree, this ancient tree is believed to have survived for some 200 million years as a species without change; individual trees have been dated at 1,000 years old. Traditional Chinese physicians used ginkgo leaves to treat asthma and chilblains; the seeds were eaten to prevent drunkenness by making alcohol unappealing, as well as for stimulating the appetite. Traditionally ginkgo has been used in tea form to enhance memory, thought processes, and brain function, and it is now being used in medications for the brain. Ginkgo is used in the treatment of senility and Alzheimer's disease as well as conditions such as ischemia, hypoxia, and impotence. All these conditions are believed to benefit from ginkgo's PAF, or platelet-activating factor, which reduces the stickiness of blood platelets. Ginkgo is also recommended for asthma, myocardial infarction, and cardiac arrhythmias, where thinner blood is beneficial. *Ginkgo biloba* extract, or GBE, is commercially available and is used to increase blood flow to the brain, combat memory loss, and treat head injuries. In clinical trials it has been shown to be effective in treating Raynaud's disease and in promoting otic blood flow, which relieves dizziness associated with inner-ear disorders. Ginkgo is just beginning to enjoy a popular following in the United States. In Europe, where it is sold in many forms, including as an intravenous drug, its prescription sales have reached some $500 million a year.

GINSENG. Korean ginseng is *Panax ginseng*, Siberian ginseng is *Eleutherococcus senticosus*, and other ginsengs are known by other scientific names. American ginseng, *Panax quinquefolium*, is a five-lobed leaf plant valued by Native Americans as a general tonic and natural restorative and adaptogen. It contains active ingredients that are prescribed for stress, insomnia, poor appetite, nervousness, and restlessness. As with all the ginsengs, the root is the part used by herbalists. Ginseng is not a fast-acting remedy, as some persons believe, but slowly helps the body increase immunity and disease resistance and fight off metabolic disturbances and the effects of chronic diseases. Although it is used in tea, tincture, or elixir form as a pick-me-up to provide energy and stimulate the central nervous system, its greatest healing value comes from long-term use.

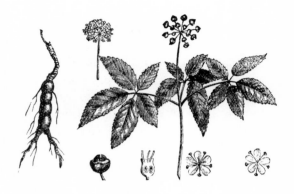

Ginseng

Because of its long history of medicinal use, ginseng is possibly the most widely recognized medicinal plant. *Panax* comes from the Greek and means "all-healing"; it is also the root of the word "panacea," or cure-all. Today ginseng is valued for its stress-reducing or adaptogenic qualities. It has an apparent general strengthening effect and helps in the treatment of neuroses, diabetes, and radiation sickness. Ginseng has been shown to promote better work and test results in students who used it regularly after taking it for an initial period to build up the body. Ginseng is believed to prevent ulcers and other stress-related conditions. Deep divers, pilots, those with impaired blood flow to the brain, and those suffering from mental debility and depression have benefited from the use of ginseng.

No real toxic effects have been shown, but some doctors caution against a possible "ginseng abuse syndrome," which is using ginseng to excess and not getting enough dietary nutrients.

GOLDENROD. *Solidago odora* and other species. This familiar yellow-flowered plant is a popular perennial in many flower gardens. Because it is so noticeable it is often mistakenly blamed for causing hay fever; actually, ragweed and other allergens cause hay fever. Sweet goldenrod was formerly listed in the U.S. Pharmacopeia and used as a carminative and mild stimulant. The leaves and/or flowers have a flavor reminiscent of anise. The tea has been taken as a beverage and as an after-dinner antacid. The Cherokees used the tea as a diaphoretic and tonic and as a treatment for colds and cough, sore mouth, and nervousness. Many tribes used it for fevers and as an anti-inflamatory. It is recommended for relieving gas and makes a gentle, effective carminative with a pleasant flavor. Goldenrod may be sold in some stores as Blue Mountain Tea.

GOLDENSEAL. *Hydrastis canadensis.* Goldenseal was one of the most important medicines of many Native Americans. The pulverized roots were used to treat eye ailments, catarrh, ulcers, and as a diuretic, laxative, and anti-inflammatory. The root was used as a wash for skin diseases and blisters, eruptions, and sores. After the Civil War goldenseal was used in so many patent medicines that the plants were nearly collected to extinction. Preparations were marketed for treatment of sciatica and rheumatic and muscular pain, and were used as an antispasmodic. It is still used in commercial eye washes, to increase cardiac output, and as an antiseptic. Although goldenseal and echinacea grow in different habitats in the wild, the two herbs are often combined in herbal preparations.

GROUND IVY. *Glechoma hederacea.* This rambling, vinelike member of the mint family is made into a tea in which the whole herb is used, or into an infusion that is used to treat lung ailments and respiratory problems. It serves as a diaphoretic and expectorant and because of its astringent properties is used externally as a wash for hemorrhoids. High in vitamin C, ground ivy is also effective in treating scurvy and other vitamin C deficiencies.

GUARANA. *Paullinia cupana.* Known as Brazilian cocoa, guarana comes from Brazil and Venezuela and is found in ethnic stores. It makes its way into medicine in the form of a paste, made from the

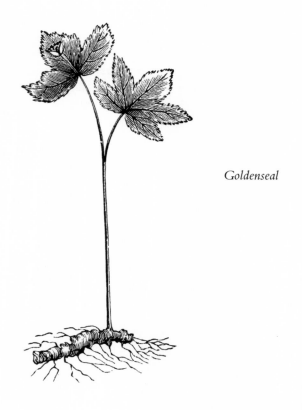

Goldenseal

pulverized, roasted seeds, which is used as a stimulant, to relieve fatigue, and in the treatment of PMS. The paste is often found in ethnic stores and some places sell it as an aphrodisiac and to relieve migraines. It is high in caffeine so should be avoided by those wishing to give up caffeine and by pregnant women. It is a natural source of theophylline, a drug used in the treatment of sleep apnea (snoring) and other breathing disorders.

HAWTHORN. *Crataegus* species. There are many varieties of hawthorn, and all their berries make excellent remedies for relieving and treating heart disease because they increase the heartbeat and eliminate palpitations. Studies show that hawthorn may dilate the arteries of the heart, thereby increasing the organ's efficiency while simultaneously increasing the strength of the beat. Hawthorn was used by Native Americans and country doctors to treat angina and to regulate heart rhythm. While nitroglycerine remains the treatment of choice for heart-failure emergencies, hawthorn berries work well as an adjunct. Some health stores stock the dried, intact berries, but others sell a standardized product of 250 mg dosage. A beneficial side effect is lowered blood pressure; the berries also have a sedative and antispasmodic effect. Hawthorn it-

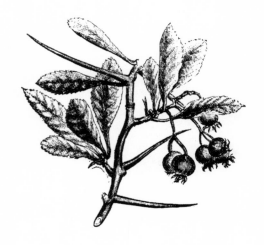

Hawthorn

self has no known negative effects when used alone in moderation, but when taken with foxglove it can be dangerous. Overuse or taking a large quantity can cause hypotension and sedation. Some persons use hawthorn leaves as a replacement for or in combination with berries when they want a lower dose of the active ingredients.

HOPS. *Humulus lupulus.* Hops flowers, used in brewing beer, are native to Europe and North America. The female flowers are called strobiles and contain chemicals that relax smooth muscle such as that found in the bowel, thereby relieving spasms and irritable bowel syndrome. Hops tea is said to improve digestion and promote sleep through a slight narcotic property. Historically, hops have been used to treat insomnia, hysteria, restlessness, and tension and to stimulate appetite. Hops have been shown to have anaphrodisiac properties that, after an initial lowering of inhibitions, cause a loss of interest in sex. Some have reported that making a sachet of hop flowers and attaching it to their pillows aids falling asleep. A standardized extract is given in a dose of 100 mg per day, but I have successfully made a sleep-inducing tea from dried leaves, flowers, or a combination of the tea in the proportion of one ounce of herb per quart of water.

Hops vines are easily grown, but will grow rampantly and will quickly choke out other garden plants, even covering a house in a single season.

HOREHOUND. *Marrubium vulgare.* This member of the mint family is found growing wild throughout Europe and is also an escaped garden plant in this country (it was originally cultivated but now grows in the wild). Horehound is a well-known expectorant and ingredient in many cough remedies. Some studies suggest that the active ingredient marrubin may influence bile secretion. A bitter

Horehound Cough Remedy

1 tablespoon dried horehound leaves, cut up
1 tablespoon lemon juice
1 cup cold water
½ cup honey or maple syrup
1 tablespoon bourbon whiskey

Boil horehound and water in an enamel or glass pan for five minutes, covered. Let stand 15 minutes or until cool. Strain into a mixture of the honey, lemon juice, and whiskey. Shake well and store in a dark place. Take by tablespoonfuls as needed for coughs and sore throats.

tea made from the leaves steeped in boiling water stimulates digestion, reduces fever, and in many women promotes menstruation.
The tea may be sweetened by adding honey and lemon. In large
doses horehound tea is an effective vermifuge.

Horehound Cough Drops

2 tablespoons dried horehound, crushed or cut up
powdered sugar
2 cups water
2 cups dark brown sugar

Boil water and horehound for 30 minutes and strain. Combine liquid and brown sugar and bring to a boil. Simmer the
syrup until it forms a hard ball when dropped into cold water. Pour into a buttered baking dish. Cool and cut into small
squares. Roll in powdered sugar and store until needed.

HORESERADISH. *Armoracia rusticana, A. lapathifolia.* Though
used most often as a condiment or as a cooking ingredient, horseradish has also been used as a diuretic and as a diaphoretic. Sweating, whether induced in a sweat lodge or sauna or by the chemical
actions of astimulant herbs such as horseradish, raises the body's
metabolic rate and is believed to cleanse, remove toxins, and promote healing.

Brought from southeastern Europe via Britain, horseradish was
used in making cold medicines during the colonial period. Debra
Stark, who owns and operates a restaurant called the Natural
Gourmet in Concord, Massachusetts, includes this recipe in her
book, *Round-the-World Cooking at the Natural Gourmet:*

Debra's Famous Cold Remedy

1 cup raw honey
1 to 2 tablespoons cayenne pepper
1 to 2 teaspoons prepared horseradish

Place honey in a glass jar. Add pepper and horseradish. Stir until liquidy. This makes enough medicine to kill many colds. Store cold remedy in the refrigerator until you feel something coming on or have a sore throat.

"This remedy works!" writes Debra. "My son, Adam, says I used to torture him with it when he was too little to appreciate its effectiveness. My brother, Daniel, took it on a bike trip to Nova Scotia and said it saved his vacation. If your throat hurts too much to swallow, this will act like balm. When you use this remedy, take a $\frac{1}{16}$-teaspoon dose or just a tiny dot. True, you will feel the heat and may think you are dying, but the honey will coat the throat, and the red pepper will warm it and stop the hurt. We all know that horseradish opens blocked passages. Cayenne pepper is rich in vitamin C, higher even than orange juice."

There are a few other very specific uses for horseradish as herbal medicine. When a small foreign body like dust is irritating the eye and can't be accessed by other means, massive tearing can be induced by smelling freshly ground or prepared horseradish. Horseradish can also be used much like smelling salts to awaken someone from a faint or to test the level of consciousness.

HORSETAIL. *Equisetum arvense.* Horsetail, also called horsetail grass, consists of bunches of tubular leafless stems. It grows in moist soils and is one of the oldest living plants. Horsetail is a tremendous source of silica and has historically been used in the treatment of hair, skin, and nail deficiencies and disorders, to stop bleeding, and to treat stomach ulcers, enlarged prostate, and cystitis. Since horsetail contains large quantities of silicon, it is also important in developing bone and cartilage and in eliminating the effects of aging on the tissues. Because it also contains saponins, horsetail acts as a diuretic and is used in treatment of kidney stones, enuresis, nephritis, and bleeding ulcers.

A standardized product is available and 1.5 grams per day of the dried herb is recommended, but the wild plant can be harvested and dried. Because of its drying properties, it has been useful in lotions used to wash sores and abscesses and to keep the feet from sweating by reducing the skin's moisture content. Acotanic acid, present in horsetail, stops secretions, including those of bleeding ulcers.

HYDRANGEA. *Hydrangea arborescens.* This native herb, a wild hydrangea, is known as seven barks to the Cherokees and other Native Americans because when the root is cut it appears to have seven layers. The root bark was dried and made into a tea for the treatment of urinary complaints, from cystitis to kidney stones. It is a powerful diuretic and is used in some commercially available back and kidney pills. Wild hydrangea grows in much of the United States and resembles the garden plant of the same name.

HYSSOP. *Hyssopus officinalis.* This mint came originally from Eurasia but has naturalized to much of this country; it is seen as a perennial shrub in the wild and as an aromatic herb in the garden. Hyssop is most widely known as a treatment for respiratory complaints including bronchitis and other inflammations of the chest and throat.

Hyssop

Today the crushed leaves are also used for cuts and bruises, and leaf infusions are applied to rheumatic joints to relieve pain. It contains marrubin, the same expectorant found in horehound, and is effective as a carminative. Some sources refer to hyssop as the biblical antiseptic because it is mentioned in so many places in the Good Book.

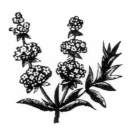

Hyssop

INDIGO. *Indigofera tinctoria.* The leaves and twigs of this shrub from Europe and South America, which produce a blue dye, have been used as a tea to treat hemorrhoids and insect bites. It is a member of the legume family and should not be confused with wild indigo of North American origin, another dye plant (see next entry). In traditional Mexican medicine, it is called *jiguilete* and is used to treat epilepsy and indigestion. Powdered indigo seeds are dusted over the body to destroy lice and to heal sores and ulcers, both here and in Mexico.

INDIGO, WILD. *Baptisia tinctoria.* Some Native Americans used the roots of this plant, made into a poultice, to treat cancer; others used the roots to make an emetic and, in weak infusions, a febrifuge and tonic. It was also used to treat diarrhea and amoebic dysentery and to reduce the swelling in tonsillitis.

IPECAC. *Cephalis ipecacuanha.* This herb is familiar to most readers because for generations, syrup of ipecac has been a standard ingredient in medicine cabinets; it promotes vomiting after a poisoning. Ipecac is also used in many cough remedies as an expectorant and stimulant. Today it is perhaps most frequently used to induce vomiting after a drug overdose. Gentler emetics are generally used for children.

IRISH MOSS. *Chondrus crispus.* Also known as carrageenan, this seaweed is used as a demulcent in battling coughs and bronchitis. It is often boiled to make a decoction or infusion, drunk as a beverage, or eaten as a vegetable. It is also effective in soothing the irritation that accompanies urinary tract and bladder infections.

JALAP. *Ipomoea jalapa.* The tuberous roots of this Mexican relative of the morning glory are used to produce jalap resins and extracts, a substance taken in small doses as a cathartic or purgative, often in combination with some carminative to prevent abdominal pain and cramping.

JERUSALEM ARTICHOKE. *Helianthus tuberosus.* The western American Indians brewed a tea from the stalks and leaves of Jerusalem artichoke or ate the flowers for rheumatism, but it is most commonly known for the use of its tubers as a winter source of food for the eastern Indians. This native sunflower with large knobby roots is a source of inulin, which the body can convert to insulin, and thus it is an important nutrient for diabetics. Since Jerusalem artichoke lacks starch, it is often substituted for potatoes in the diet. Its name comes from a corruption of the French *girasol,* which means "turn to the sun." In the South, particularly in the Appalachians, the roots are simply called artichokes or hearti-chokes. They may be found today in grocery stores as "sunchokes" and are easy to establish in the garden. But beware, they may be-come a pest in one or two seasons, as they are invasive. The tubers dried and pounded can be chewed to relieve a sore throat.

JEWELWEED. *Impatiens capensis* or *I. biflora.* The native American impatiens has provided much relief from insect stings, sunburn, and dermatitis associated with poison oak and ivy. I have personally used it to treat nettle stings in soldiers, a yellow jacket sting in my nephew, and poison ivy rashes in dozens of individuals. Jewelweed is so called because when the plant is immersed in water, it shines silver like a mirrored surface and when removed the water does not cling to the leaf surfaces. It is also called spotted or pale touch-me-knot, depending on the flower color, because once the seeds are mature, the slightest jarring of the seed pod will send them flying for some distance.

Jewelweed, a common plant along sunny streams and springs and in wet meadows, is a tender annual plant that eagerly puts forth new growth as soon as spring arrives. (Many people believe that jewelweed is always found growing near poison oak or ivy, but I have not found this to be the case.) The plant may reach heights of three or four feet, even more in ideal conditions, and produces thick stands. The stems are strong and knotty, succulent and juicy. I use the whole plant when possible, though my wife breaks small branches off as needed so that the plant continues to flourish. The first hard frost marks the end of the year's jewelweed crop, but per-sons who suffer from poison ivy or similar rashes can process the plants in a blender and freeze them in ice-cube trays for winter use. I simply rub the crushed stems, leaves, and juice on the afflicted or exposed part of the bite or burn and it heals quickly, the pain stop-ping almost immediately.

Jew's Ear

The well-known herbalist James A. Duke notes that the Potawatomi Indians infused the plants for treatment of bruises, chest colds, cramps, and urticaria (hives), while the Creek Indians speeded up delivery of a baby with a warm douche made from a jewelweed infusion.

JEW'S EAR. *Auricula judea.* This is a fungus that grows on elder bushes; it was brought here by the Irish. The fungus is white on the outside and black on the inside. It has veins and its shape resembles that of an ear. The dried fungus is powdered, made into a tea, and is taken for chilblains and to reduce swelling of inflamed tonsils and throat.

JIMSONWEED. *Datura stramonium* and *D. metalloides.* This is an interesting plant to know about, but it is dangerous and unpredictable and should be used only by professionals under controlled conditions. The drug scopolamine is derived from this plant; delivered through a patch, it is used to combat motion sickness. The forerunners of the nicotine patches, these patches are marketed as Transdermal Scope and are used by the military and other government agencies.

Also commonly referred to as datura, it is one of the ingredients used in potions that greatly lower the metabolism so that one might be perceived to be dead, later returning to life. In parts of South America it is used by native healers as a painkiller during surgery; it may be found growing outside their doorway—their "shingle," so to speak.

The plant, however, has dangerous, potentially deadly, hallucinogenic properties, including giving the user a sense of being able to fly. There have been many reported cases of people plummeting to their deaths while "scoping out"; others have drowned or nearly drowned, for use of datura made them feel as if their bodies were on fire and the only way to quench it was to dive into a pool of water.

The benefits of using jimsonweed are not worth the huge risk, especially when parts of the plant are utilized in which the components cannot be measured with certainty. Its name is reportedly a corruption of the word "Jamestown," and it is said that during the Revolutionary War, the Jamestown settlers cooked it in greens to sicken the British troops occupying their homes. Other historical accounts show jimsonweed eaters naked in the snow and barking like dogs or wolves. Its other name, thornapple, refers to its mace-like seed pods, which are covered with stickers or burs.

JOE-PYE-WEED. *Eupatorium dubium* or *E. purpureum.* Possibly the only herb named after an American Indian, Joe-Pye-weed takes its name from the New England Native American who used its roots to cure white colonists of typhus and other fevers. The herbalist James A. Duke says the Algonquins used the white flowers to cure venereal diseases and used the red flowers for dysmenorrhea. Cherokees used the roots for the same purpose. A syrup is made to treat intermittent fevers.

Joe-Pye-Weed Syrup

Put three handfuls of the herb in a basin filled with about six quarts of water and let it steep until the herb is softened. Strain, add one pint of molasses or honey, and boil it down to about a pint of syrup, taking care not to burn it.

The leaves are applied as a poultice to burns, other skin sores and eruptions, and to aching joints.

JOJOBA. *Simmondsia chinensis.* The oil, which is cold-pressed from the seeds, was used topically by both Apaches and other American Southwest Indians as well as more recently by immigrants from Israel. Interestingly, the plant grows in the desert in both Israel and the American Southwest, despite their geographical distance. The seeds are toxic to humans, but the oil is used to alleviate skin conditions such as chapped lips and sunburn and is believed to stimulate hair growth and regeneration. Today the oil is being researched as an ingredient in cosmetics and hair treatments as well as industrial lubricants.

JUJUBE. *Zyzyphus jujube.* The seeds of this plant were brought to America by African slaves, who used them for purposes ranging from taking it to increase muscular strength to consuming as a nutrient to serving as an antiallergen, sedative, and antitussive. The fruits, which contain one or two seeds, have been shown to reduce ulcers and lower high blood pressure. You can find jujube in health food and ethnic stores.

JUNIPER. *Juniperus communis* and other species. Some members of the genus are called junipers, whereas others are called cedars. For example, *Juniperus virginiana,* an American species, is called the Eastern red cedar. The British used juniper berries to flavor meat in cooking as well as to flavor gin, a more commonly recognized flavor. An extracted substance, known as sabinal, is used to preserve catgut suture material, lending credence to juniper's use by herbal and native practitioners to fight infection. The needles, berries, and bark are used in steam treatment and vapor inhalation for bronchitis and chest congestion. Russian immigrants used juniper as an antibiotic by applying the oils extracted in water or alcohol.

The berries themselves, while being useful as a flavoring or medicine source, should not be ingested, as they have been considered to cause kidney damage. A commonly followed rule is to limit juniper tea consumption to two cups a day or less for no longer than six weeks at a time. The tea is good for arthritic inflammations and pain, as a diuretic and as an emmenagogue.

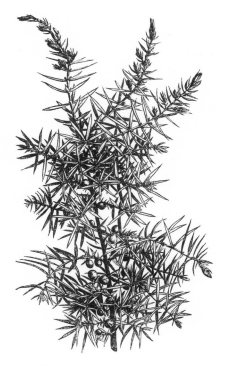

Juniper sprig with berries

If you want to grow your own juniper berries and needles, you will have to make certain that you have both male and female plants because they are separate-sex plants, so both are needed for successful pollination. Males have yellowish brown flowers and females have green flowers followed by the berries.

Elderly persons, children under two, and pregnant women should not use juniper unless a doctor tells them it is all right in their case.

Juniper Tea

1 tablespoon juniper berries
1 quart water

Bruise the berries between two spoons or in a mortar and pestle, but don't break them into little pieces; they will be hard to strain. Bring the water to a hard boil, pour over the berries, and steep for 20 minutes to half an hour. Strain.

KALMIA. *Kalmia latifolia* and other species. Kalmias include the mountain laurels and related plants with names such as lamb-kill, calfkill, and sheep laurel. Kalmia can be lethal when taken internally because it depresses the respiratory system. To relieve pain in joints, a salve or ointment is made from the leaves and applied externally to the affected area. It is said that birds that have eaten kalmia berries can poison whatever or whoever then eats them. Among American Indians, the Lumbees bathed in the irritating decoction to relieve itch, scabies, and the seven-year itch, and the Penobscots used kalmia, cedar, and salt in a poultice for sprains and strains. The herbalist Joseph Meyer says that Indians used kalmia to commit suicide, but this is suspect, since for most Native Americans, if not all, suicide was a dishonorable way to die.

KAMALA. *Mallotus philippinensis.* This herb imported from the Middle East and Africa is enjoying an increased popularity. It is most commonly used as a taenifuge, or tapeworm remedy, among members of certain religious groups who must eat animals that are raised and prepared in a special way. Kamala may also be found to be in use by military personnel who participated in the Gulf War and became aware of its use against parasites. It is also used by persons from the Indian subcontinent for the same purposes and as a purgative. The hairs and glands of the fruits are sold as either a powder or a liquid extract.

KAOLIN. This medicinal is not an herb, but it bears mentioning because many herbal formulae call for it as an ingredient. Kaolin is a mineral-laden white clay that originally was mined in China at a locality called K'ao-ling Hill. The name is now generic for other white clays of the same type found around the world and utilized in medicine; it gives the "kao-" prefix to the commercial antidiarrhea medicine Kaopectate. In some black cultures Kaolin is known as "the healing earth." I have recommended the use of white clay from riverbanks to soldiers in various military schools and in U.S. and other forces to fight dysentery, diarrhea, and dehydration. It is usually used in suspension in a liquid, but it can be eaten as clay if necessary.

KAVA KAVA. *Piper methysticum.* This South Pacific island plant has been grown and used for centuries as a relaxing herb. It is sold in health food stores in the United States and as an over-the-counter medicine in Europe in a standard dosage of 150 to 750 milligrams. The ground root is mildly psychoactive and a decoction made with it sharpens the senses while relaxing the mind and body with feelings of peace and contentment. Substances called kavalactones are the primary active ingredient.

Fiji and Guam islanders still use this remedy extensively, as do other South Pacific cultures. In this country, it is usually taken in a dosage of one to three capsules (150 to 250 mg), taken a half hour before bedtime as a sleep aid or when relief is needed from a headache.

KELP. *Laminaria* species. This giant seaweed, which may grow to 20 feet tall in giant underwater kelp forests, is powdered and used as a substitute for sea salt in the kitchen and converted to algin for use as a stabilizing agent in pharmaceutical and cosmetic products. Unlike many medicinal plants, most types of kelp actually taste good when eaten. Kelp provides many trace elements and is heartily recommended by dietitians as a source of potassium. Kelp is still used to combat obesity (it regulates the thyroid gland) and is found listed as laminaria in many herbal weight-loss formulas. Cooked kelp soothes mucous membranes irritated by sore throat or vomiting. It also serves to purify the blood and act as an alterative, gradually returning the patient to normal health. Native Americans used it for the prevention and treatment of "big neck," or goiter, and modern research has found kelp to be high in iodine, which proves its value for this purpose.

Virtually all health food stores and supplement catalogs offer several forms of kelp. Today kelp is used in all treatments of iodine deficiency and in heavy-metal poisoning prophylaxis and treatment. It has also been proven to interfere with the growth of some bacteria and may promote weight loss if there is abnormal functioning of the thyroid gland. Researchers working for the former

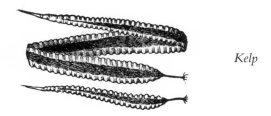

Kelp

Atomic Energy Commission found in animal experiments that consumption of kelp helped prevent absorption of radioactive substances, especially strontium-90.

Kelp Tea

2 to 3 teaspoons dried kelp frond
1 cup boiling water

Pour boiling water over powdered, dried kelp frond and drink after a 10-minute steeping period.

KINNIKINNICK. *Arctostaphylos uva-ursi. Uva-ursi* is Algonquin for "bear grape," but this plant is more commonly called bearberry. Many prefer to hang on to the Native American name, and kinnikinnick is often sold at pow wows both as a medicinal plant and as an ingredient in smoking mixtures. The fresh leaves are gathered in late fall and early winter, dried, and pulverized. The infusion is used for treating urinary problems in both sexes and for urinary incontinence in women.

This evergreen shrub grows about six inches high and is found in coniferous forests from New Jersey and Pennsylvania westward to California, Colorado, and Utah as well as other southwestern states. The herbalist Charles Millspaugh (who describes the Native Americans as "American aborigines") has this to say about kinnikinnick: "Should we prescribe on the palliative principle, and at the same time believe in disinfection by killing germs, I could barely point to a drug more adapted to diseases of the kidney, bladder, and urethra."

KNAPWEED. *Centaurea nigra.* Also called black knapweed in Britain, where it was traditionally used as a tonic and as a diuretic and diaphoretic, it is known in some places as star thistle and is a relative of our thistles. It can be grown here in the States, but is often imported. The herb is made into a tea or decoction and has a bitter taste.

KNOTWEED. *Polygonum aviculare* and *P. cuspidatum.* Also known as nine joints and pigweed, this member of the buckwheat family grows close to the ground. Its leaves are attached directly to the main stem and there are knots along the stems. Knotweed should not be confused with other members of the buckwheat family, because eating raw knotweed can cause stomach disturbances. It is native to North America but grows in Europe as well. Though science has yet to confirm knotweed's use as an astringent or antidiarrheal, these uses make sense, owing to the high tannin content. Some Native Americans used a tea of knotweed as a remedy for gallstones; it has also been used as a styptic and to stop nosebleed, by crushing it and applying the juice.

KOLA NUT. *Cola acuminata.* This herb, which originated in Africa, is widely grown in the tropics today and is sold separately or in combination with other herbs as a stimulant, to relieve headaches (including those from coffee withdrawal), migraines, and in preparations to prevent sleepiness. Of course, its widest usage is in sodas. Cola drinks account for nearly three quarters of the soft drink market. Kola arrived in this country during the Civil War, when it was prescribed for treating depression and taken to prepare for severe mental or physical exertion—today's definition of a stimulant. We now also know that it is a diuretic. Some asthmatic persons enjoy relief from constricted air passages after taking kola tea or cola beverages. The *Journal of the American Medical Association* has recommended cola drinks to help manage childhood asthma.

Kola nuts in the raw form are the seeds of this tree; the seedling leaves are also used and may be bought in a dried or powdered form. Kola is approximately 10 percent caffeine, so persons who have been told to avoid caffeine should not use kola nut in any form. Excessive use of kola nut or cola products can result in insomnia, stomach upset, including cramps, and increased irritability or moodiness.

Kola Tea

1 to 2 teaspoons kola powder
1 cup boiling water

Simmer the kola powder or nuts in the boiling water for 10 minutes. Take 1 cup three times a day for headaches and as a pick-me-up. Sugar or other sweeteners may be added to taste.

KOMBUCHA. Though popularly known today as Manchurian mushroom or Kombucha mushroom, this unique organism is not a mushroom at all. Instead, it is a form created by the symbiotic relationship between certain yeasts of the *Saccharomyces* genus and bacteria of the acetobacter species and acetic bacteria like xylinium and gluconicum. It creates a "mother" organism, which reproduces itself in about 10 days time in the proper environment of sugar and tea water. A vinegar is produced and drunk in various amounts for treatment of liver and blood toxification and skin conditions, and to fight the aging process. Although the Kombucha organism is believed to help stimulate the immune system, it is recommended that persons with immune deficiencies such as AIDS not use it at all.

Kombucha's greatest benefits seem to be in helping the liver do its job of detoxifying the body, in fighting allergic responses and in some cases, helping the body lose cellulite. It is also believed that excessive use could lead to fatal liver diseases, so the jury is still out on this latest herbal weapon to gain widespread attention. Some believe that the "baby" Kombucha must be passed on without charge, while some health stores have been found selling them for $50 or more.

KUDZU. *Pueraria lobata.* The powdered form of this herb's root was used by Chinese herbalists as a cancer-preventive agent, but it is most commonly known for its use as a starch. The flour is used in Oriental cooking much as cornstarch is used here and is an ingredient in many prepared Chinese foods. In capsule form, the starch also serves as an effective vehicle for other herbs. Today, researchers at Harvard Medical School believe that it can effectively eliminate a desire for alcohol. Their experiments were done with hamsters, but it has been used to treat alcoholism in China and Japan for centuries, where it is sold over the counter in pill form. A tea is made from the powdered kudzu and drunk in China. In American experiments one active ingredient of kudzu was isolated, synthesized, and then patented as diadzin. But diadzin is not the only key to kudzu's effectiveness, because the original chemical was changed (synthesized) in the lab.

L

LADY'S SLIPPER. *Cypripedium calceolus.* Lady's slipper is an American wild orchid and is protected in most places. At one time, it was known as American valerian and the root was prescribed for a wide variety of emotional problems, as a hypnotic, and for epilepsy and neuralgia. Many country doctors might have prescribed a boiled extract of the roots as a sedative or to treat hysteria. Some Indians used it for female problems and others used it for tuberculosis. In large doses, it can cause hallucinations and giddiness. It is generally avoided today.

LAVENDER. *Lavandula officinalis.* This plant is known as an antiemetic, which means that it will stop vomiting, but it should be used with care because lavender oil can be poisonous. An infusion made from the flowers is taken internally as an antispasmodic or as a sedative, and to cure menstrual cramps. A liniment or salve is

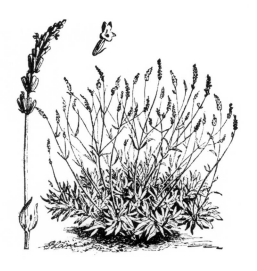

Lavender

made from the flowers or oil, which is used externally to stimulate the nerve endings. Some herbalists used distilled oil on the forehead to cure headache and to relieve depression or the doldrums. Others make "dream pillows" stuffed with lavender flowers; some find that smelling them promotes sound sleep and pleasant dreams. The tea made from lavender flowers has a carminative effect.

LEMONGRASS. *Cymbopogon citratus.* Historically, a tea made from lemongrass has been used as a treatment for managing nervous and gastrointestinal disorders. Some sources say that it is the most popular plant used in traditional South American medicine, and it is widely used in herbal medicine in this country. The country doctor might have used it to reduce fevers, but scientific studies call it a very effective placebo, finding no chemicals that can be isolated or synthesized.

LICORICE. *Glycrrhiza glabra.* The root of this vine, a member of the pea family, has been used for centuries both as a sweetener and as a medicinal herb in the treatment of ulcers and stomach problems, in hypoglycemia, and for cirrhosis and other liver damage. Since licorice has displayed anti–inflammatory activity and demulcent properties, as well as a natural sweetness, it has been used in cough syrups and in treating ulcers. Excessive consumption of licorice can lead to sodium and water retention and potassium depletion. Taken in moderation, this herb is generally considered to have benefits that outweigh its possible dangers. It has been used to treat cancer in many countries and cultures.

American country doctors in the 1800s used licorice to treat urinary tract problems, chest congestion, and tuberculosis, as well as to mask the bitterness of other herbs. It also might have been used in Native American treatments for earache and constipation. The influence of the Chinese would have prompted its use in treating cirrhosis and hepatitis. Its antifungal properties make licorice effective when either taken internally or used as a wash for yeast infections, candida, and streptococcal and staphylococcal infections.

Persons using licorice should be aware of the possibility of electrolyte imbalances—which can be reversed with potassium replacements (eating a banana)—or the possibility of hypertension and edema.

LIFE ROOT. *Senecio aureus.* This is also known as squaw weed (as are many other herbs), false valerian, and coughweed. Life root, a perennial member of the aster family, grows in swamps in the eastern and central United States. It was used widely by Native Americans in the treatment of childbirth pains and to hasten the onset of labor, and is found today in some commercial preparations used for these same purposes. It can cause abortion in some cases and therefore should be used only by professionals.

LINDEN. *Tilia* species. These trees produce odd-shaped flower structures that are infused or decocted to produce a demulcent tea for relief of inflamed mucous membranes, particularly sore throats. The flowers are brewed as a tranquilizer and as a bedtime beverage to promote sound sleep. They may be sold or offered under the names lime, linden, or basswood, and in some Spanish stores under the name *tilia*.

LOVAGE. *Levisticum officinale.* This plant, a member of the parsley family, has long been known to be effective in treating gas problems—colic, flatulence, and intestinal and stomach cramps. Introduced from Europe, this perennial plant has escaped; it grows wild in much of the West and South and has been found as far west as New Mexico. As with any member of the parsley family, it is essential when gathering from the wild not to mistakenly pick its dangerous relative, poison hemlock. Known to some herbalists as love-parsley, lovage's only romantic benefit is in providing sweet breath. Tea made from the root has been recommended as a diuretic and as an emmenagogue, but there is no scientific evidence to support its efficacy for this.

LUFFA. *Luffa cylindrica.* The most common use for luffa sponges or luffa gourds in this country is as scrubbers in the bath, and for washing dishes. However, for centuries luffa has been used in Chinese medicine in decoction form. The leaves and immature fruits are boiled and the water used to promote blood circulation, break up fever, and discharge phlegm as well as to treat swollen testes, hemorrhoids, and bellyaches. To address back pain and arthritis, ½ ounce of green luffa is cut up and boiled in one pint water until the liquid is reduced to half. This is strained and taken once daily. Luffa is known as Chinese okra when eaten as an immature vegetable. The mature gourds are burned in a sealed container to produce charcoal, which is mixed with a 1:1 alcohol-water solution to form a paste. This is rubbed on herpetic rashes and relieves pain when prescription drugs are ineffective.

MAGNOLIA. *Magnolia grandifolia, M. virginia,* other species. This tree is associated with antebellum Southern plantations in America, but it is also found in other parts of the United States and the world. In Asian medicine the flowers are made into a tea used to treat headache, stuffy nose, and a hot face and head because it is believed that the tea dissipates heat and alleviates pain. Chinese herbalists call magnolia *hsin-i* or *mu-pi* and call the bark *ch'uan-huo-po.* In Mexican medicine the magnolia is known as *flor de corazon,* or flower of the heart, no doubt in part in tribute to the romantic fragrance of its blossoms—but some herbalists do recommend drinking a blossom tea to strengthen the heart. The bark was ground into a powder by the ancient Aztecs and later by the Mexicans and was used to make a tea that promoted heart stimulation. The Aztec name *yoloxochitl* also means "heart flower."

Chinese herbalists and doctors specify magnolia bark for various stomach disorders including gastritis, nausea, abdominal swelling and distention, and for asthma, coughs, colds, and diarrhea.

The Aztecs also used magnolia bark tea for senility and in the treatment of mental stupor, conditions now attributed to Alzheimer's disease. Today, some American herbalists drink the tea cold when they desire tobacco, with some positive results.

Other sources recommend using a liquid extract as a diaphoretic and a stimulant.

MA HUANG. *See* Ephedra.

MALE FERN. *Dryopterix filix-mas.* This fern grows one to three feet tall from a creeping rhizome and is found from coast to coast and border to border. Under each toothed leaflet can be found spore capsules with either kidney-shaped or round shields (good to know when you're trying to locate or identify this plant in the wild). The rhizomes are gathered for medicinal use; until 1965 they were listed in the U.S. Pharmacopeia as the most potent treatment for tapeworms available. A substance known as oleoresin paralyzes the tapeworm so that it releases its grip on the bowel and can be discharged. The remedy is also effective for animals.

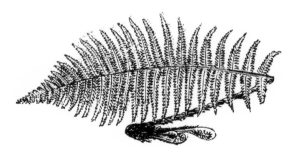

Male fern

Male Fern Tea for Tapeworms
1 to 2 teaspoons ground or powdered male fern root
1 pint water
½ teaspoon salt

Simmer all ingredients about 20 minutes and cool. Drink
by the tablespoonful, waiting two hours between doses for
effect. Works best when fats and oils have been removed
from the diet for three days prior to treatment.

Male fern should not be used in conjunction with castor oil because the oil retains the fern's toxin in the body too long and may
produce negative side effects.

MALLOW. *Malva neglecta, M. sylvestris.* This plant is also known as
the cheese plant, owing to the shape of its seed pods, or fruits,
which look like cheese wheels. Native and folk healers have prescribed the gelatinous tea made by boiling the leaves, fruits, and
roots for treatment of irritations and inflammations of the gastrointestinal tract, from the throat to the rectum. The demulcent properties have brought relief to irritated kidneys and bladders as well.
The leaves are made into a poultice and used against irritations
of the skin such as insect stings, abrasions, sunburn, and thermal
burns. Mexican Americans have used the flowers as relief for
toothache by placing the chewed petals against the offending tooth.
Drinking mallow tea has been found to relieve the difficult speech
and painful swallowing caused by swollen tonsils. The leaves can be
dried for later use.

MANDRAKE, AMERICAN. *See* Mayapple.

MAPLE. *Acer rubrum* and other species. About one cup of dried red maple inner bark is boiled in one quart of water and, when cooled, applied to swollen, puffy eyes for relief. Maple sap, mostly from the sugar maple, is reduced by boiling it without scorching it to make maple syrup, which can be used as a sweetener in making other medicines or cough syrups. It takes approximately 30 gallons of sap to make one gallon of syrup.

MARIGOLD. *Calendula officinalis.* Now known as pot marigold (*calendula* to Mexicans), this herb has long been used in salves, tinctures, infusions, and decoctions. In lotions it is applied externally as a treatment for sore, dry nipples; for rashes, including diaper and heat rash; and for burns from sun or scald. Tinctures and teas are taken internally as antihemorrhagics and to relieve ulcers and other gastric disorders. A poultice made from the leaves is effective in reducing calluses when applied regularly. In culinary circles, pot marigold is used to color rice yellow in place of the more expensive saffron, and the edible flowers are now popular as a garnish in dipping vegetable plates and salads.

MARIJUANA. *Cannabis sativa.* Hardly needing a description, this illegal herb has been used in many societies for treatment of glaucoma and other optic disorders where reduction of ocular pressure is important. It has also been smoked for relief from the suffering of both cancer and cancer treatments, sleep disorders, and pain. Several states have recognized the healing properties of marijuana and have declared it legal for medical purposes with a doctor's permission. Chinese records show its use for more than 2,000 years and Native Americans make mention of it in tea form to relieve bronchial ailments. It is effective as an antispasmodic, and some herbalists have mixed it with horehound for a tea to treat coughing spells. Poultices have been used to draw out carbuncles and boils as well as embedded splinters and other foreign material.

MARJORAM. *Origanum vulgare.* This member of the mint family is best known for its use in flavoring fish and meat dishes. It is often known as sweet marjoram, to distinguish it from its relative, Greek marjoram, or oregano, which is more pungent. Marjoram oil was prescribed for toothaches in medieval Europe and is still found to be an effective remedy. In Mexican medicine it is known as *mejorana*, which means "gets better" or "better maker," and is popular as a tea to alleviate stomachache, cramps, and nausea. It is also effective as a carminative and has some diuretic qualities. Poultices wrapped around the throat are used for treating sore throats and swollen glands. Marjoram will probably be drawing more attention in the future, as extracts have been shown to have antioxidant properties, a quality that is currently a popular component in the treatment of many ailments and conditions.

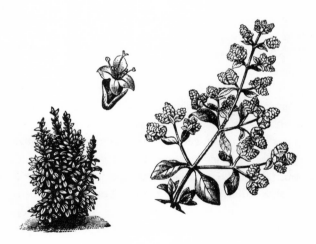

Marjoram

MARSHMALLOW. *Althaea offinalis.* The marshmallow is closely related to the cheese plants or mallows. The genus name, *Althaea*, comes from a Greek verb that means "to heal." The entire plant contains the mucilage that soothes mucous membranes. Some druggists still sell the root, which is used to make a cough syrup. It can also be gathered fresh.

Marshmallow Cough Syrup

1 cup peeled, chopped marshmallow roots, stems, and leaves
1 cup orange juice
1 pint water
½ cup honey

Boil the marshmallow until the water is reduced by half and mucilage is released. Strain, if desired, and mix with honey and orange juice. Take a full tablespoon to relieve irritated throat and stop cough.

Marshmallow (and other mallows) can be used to make a soothing wash for the tender gums of teething infants. Similarly, the mushy, overcooked pods of marshmallow's relative okra can be used for the same purpose; just rub the gums with them.

After having been introduced from Europe, marshmallow now grows wild in much of North America, mainly in damp places including salt marshes. It was used originally to make the candy known by the same name. Okra, rose of Sharon bushes, and other members of this plant's extensive family, Malvaceae, also contain beneficial mucilaginous properties.

MARSH MARIGOLD. *Caltha palustris.* In some wild food guides this plant is called cowslip because elk cows (*and* bulls) enjoy its taste. It is mentioned here with a warning that the raw leaves can cause heart arrhythmias, severe gastric convulsions, and blistering of the skin. However, they may be useful in removing warts when the caustic sap is carefully squeezed onto them drop by drop.

Historically, marsh marigold was used in various forms by Native Americans. For example, the Ojibwas boiled the crushed plant with maple syrup as a cough syrup and the Eskimos used the leaf to make a tea as a laxative.

MATE. *Ilex paraguayensis.* Herbalists encounter mate in commercial teas with names like Morning Thunder, so named because of its caffeine content. Mate comes from the South American holly tree also known as *yerba mate* (pronounced mah-tay) and contains vitamin C as well as caffeine, which makes this herb nutritious as well as stimulating. It is said that gauchos, South American cowboys, live on meat and mate. A six-ounce cup of mate contains 50 milligrams of caffeine, a little less than coffee. Mate's diuretic properties make it useful in alleviating the bloating of PMS. Persons with esophageal cancer are advised to avoid mate.

MAYAPPLE. *Podophyllum peltatum.* Although used commercially in various anticancer and other medicines, the entire green mayapple plant is considered toxic except for the ripe fruits, which are also known as raccoon berries. Because of the extremely violent nature of the intestinal purgative effects and its impact on the nervous system, it is recommended that the herbalist avoid medications containing mayapple, also known as American mandrake. Even a tiny amount of dried mayapple root powder is an extremely powerful laxative.

The synthetic drugs Etoposide and Tenopiside are derivatives of the naturally occurring chemical podophyllotoxin (which is extracted from mayapple) and have proved effective antitumor agents.

Mint

MESQUITE. *Prosopis juliflora.* In the southwestern United States, the sap is extracted from mesquite and boiled in water to make a cure for dysentery. While in Texas, I learned that the water from boiling the mesquite beans (a long process) also works well for treating diarrhea. A decoction made from beans, bark, and root is effective in soothing irritated bowels and intestines. The leaves are used to make a wash for soothing irritated eyes.

MILK THISTLE. *Silybum marianum.* The name may come from the fact that many European wet nurses included milk thistle in their diets in the belief that the cooked leaves increased lactation. Native to the Mediterranean area but naturalized in the United States, milk thistle is the source of silymarin, which is used in liver regeneration. It is also a component in treating liver damage caused by alcohol abuse and mushroom poisoning, particularly cases involving the amanitas. Milk thistle is now harvested and prepared commercially by methyl alcohol extraction, evaporation, and collection of the powder; a standard dose is 300 to 600 milligrams per day. It is used in the treatment of jaundice, psoriasis, the liver, and menstrual difficulties, as well as varicose veins and heavy-metal poisoning.

MINT. *Mentha* species. There are too many varieties of mint to name each one here. In Mexico and the American Southwest mint is known as *hierba buena*, or the "good herb." It is such a good cure-all that my wife has said, "When I get sick on the stomach, I'm like a cat. I go out in the yard and eat some mint." Once, during a car trip, she settled her upset stomach (brought on by car sickness) by eating some wild mint I found along a creek. Pennyroyal mint has been used as an emmenagogue to induce menstruation and as an insect repellant. All the mints tend to be antiemetic and are used in traditional as well as commercial preparations for relief of gas, upset stomach, air and seasickness, and morning sickness symptoms. Mint tea is a mild stimulant but it also is used to calm an upset

Mistletoe

stomach and promote a sound sleep. Mint leaves in the bath promote calming of the nerves and aid in falling asleep.

Country doctors found American Indians putting native mints to work in the treatment of bronchial disorders, including pneumonia, stomach distress, and menstrual discomforts.

Menthol is the distillate of mint oil and is effective when used in vapor treatment or inhalation therapy for relieving nasal, sinus, and chest congestion. Herbalists can make their own salves and creams with mint if they wish, but its healing and painkilling properties are available in such over-the-counter medications as Solarcaine, Unguentine, and Ben-Gay.

Mint is easy to grow, often becoming invasive and functioning as a healthy weed.

MISTLETOE. *Viscum album.* This is the European mistletoe, classified in the United Kingdom as a drug available only through pharmacists, which differs from American mistletoe. Experimentation with both is discouraged, although historically they have been used in cardiac and high blood pressure medicines, and as a sedative and antispasmodic. European mistletoe works on the central nervous system and therefore should be used only by professionals.

MOTHERWORT. *Leonurus cardiaca.* This member of the mint family has been used successfully as an antispasmodic in tea form and as an emmenagogue.

MUGWORT. *Artemesia vulgaris.* Flower heads and dried leaves of mugwort are used to make a tea for treating various female disorders, including menopausal difficulties and painful menstruation. The tea, one ounce of herb to a pint of water, should be administered 10 to 12 days before menstruation is expected to begin and continue through the menstrual period. Pregnant women are urged to refrain from its use because it can cause uterine contractions, which may in turn cause a miscarriage. The tea is also said to stimulate appetite, ease childbirth, and induce sweating.

MULLEIN. *Verbascum thapsus.* This is a unique medicinal plant in that the dried leaves used to treat asthma and bronchitis are smoked either in a pipe or in cigarette form. Known in Latin America as *gordolobo*, or fatleaf, it is used to treat bronchial disorders and other problems, such as discouraging bedwetting by thickening urine and keeping it in the body longer.

Bedwetting Tea

½ teaspoon ground mullein
⅛ teaspoon sugar
¼ cup water

Soak sugar and mullein in water for 1 to 2 hours and administer before bedtime.

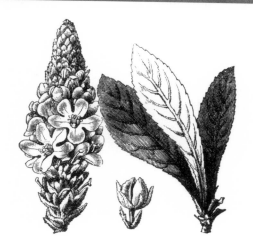

Mullein

I have made a highly effective earache medicine by placing two handfuls of mullein flowers in a pint of olive oil and exposing the mixture to the sun for 10 days to two weeks. This oil was then strained and daubed in the outer ear of a cranky child, weary adult, and others.

John Gerrard, the famous early English herbalist, said that mullein flowers are also good for treating piles; his preparation method was unusual in that he put the flowers in oil and then used the heat of warm, decaying dung heaps to keep the concoction warm and make extraction of the active ingredients possible. Paradoxically, mullein leaves have been smoked to treat asthma because mullein relaxes the bronchial tubes, allowing breathing to return to normal.

MUSTARD. *Brassica nigra.* Ground mustard seeds mixed with lard have long been used to alleviate pain, particularly in joints, to relieve chest pain in bronchial disorders, and to relieve cold and flu symptoms when added to footbaths. When applying mustard plasters, caution must be used to prevent damage to skin by blistering and burning. To make a mustard plaster, mix ground mustard seeds or powdered mustard (known as flowers of mustard in some stores) with flour and water into a paste. Wrap the paste in a damp cloth or leaves and place on the back or chest of a person suffering with cold, flu, or other bronchial disorders.

NEEM. *Azadirachta indica.* This large evergreen tree grown in India produces seeds from which oil is extracted and used as a contraceptive; infusions are made from the roots and bark for treating malaria and from the leaves for treating worms. The oils are available in health and herb stores. Persons using it for skin conditions, ulcers, and cardiovascular ailments should be aware of possible contraception as a side effect.

NETTLE. *Urtica dioica.* Stinging nettle is a good name for this herb, which has relatives in Europe and the Americas. Its well-known stinging effect comes from barbs in tiny cells that fire a dose of formic acid into the skin when touched. The Aztecs used this plant, which they called *ortiga mayor*, to reduce hemorrhage and nosebleed, and it is still used for the same purposes today. For nosebleed, a wad of cotton or paper is dipped in expressed nettle juice and placed in the nostril; nettle juice can be expressed by squeezing the stalks in a blender or by pounding them with mortar and pestle. Cooked nettles are a traditional food in many countries and are very nutritious.

The entire plant is used. Taken internally, cooked nettles and nettle tea are used to control bleeding ulcers or excessive menstrual flow. Nettle is used as a diuretic and as a tonic, being high in chlorophyll. In some countries and stores in this country, it is the main ingredient in a product marketed as chlorophyll tea.

The sting of nettle is used in the treatment of gouty arthritis, much like the Asian practice of allowing bees to sting a swollen joint. Research has shown dried nettles in capsules to relieve allergy and hay fever symptoms. An infusion is suggested for the same purpose. Nettle's diuretic properties make it useful in managing congestive heart failure and high blood pressure. Nettles contain substances that mobilize uric acid from joints and eliminate it from the body, which reduces pain, swelling, and sore joints.

Nettle tea is used externally to shrink and reduce inflammation of hemorrhoids. Also, the seeds are soaked in water and the water used as a rinse to add luster to the hair after shampooing.

To avoid being stung when harvesting stinging nettles, one should handle them with gloves or tongs.

NIGHT-BLOOMING CEREUS. *Selenicereus grandiflorus.* The country doctor may have run across accounts of how the green part of this cactus from the West Indies was traditionally used as a cardiac stimulant and tonic. Traditional use includes taking in the active ingredient, cactine; it is reported to have a similar effect on the heart as digitalis, and should therefore be considered dangerous.

NUTMEG. *Myristica fragrans.* Much of our nutmeg now comes from the West Indies, but this herb is a native of New Guinea. The seed is used as a cooking spice, but in medicine it serves as a carminative, being used to relieve nausea and vomiting and to treat indigestion and diarrhea. Excessive consumption can lead to intoxication, sedation, and rapid heartbeat.

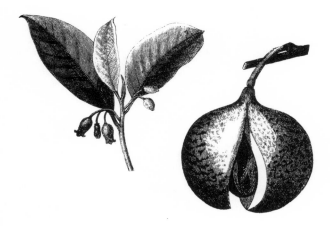

Nutmeg

OAK. *Quercus* species. Sometimes marketed as tanner's bark, oak bark, which is astringent, is used to reduce hemorrhoids, dry poison ivy and poison oak rashes or burns, and treat diarrhea and dysentery. It is also used as a gargle for throat problems. All oak bark contains tannin or tannic acid, and thus care should be exercised when it is taken internally because excess use can cause kidney damage. It is known as *encina* in Mexico, and the leaves are macerated into a poultice for application to insect stings and bites and to stop itching. Oak bark infusion is also used as a douche to fight yeast infections.

OATS. *Avena sativa.* Also known as groats, the rolled or flattened oat seeds are used in medicine as a nutritive because they are a good source of fiber and are easily digested. They are used externally to treat skin conditions, including burns and rashes from

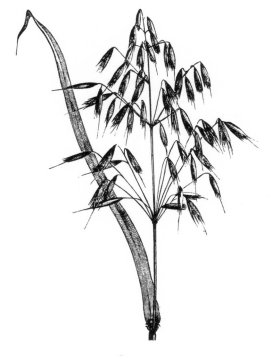

Oats

plants and insects. Oat is also employed in preparations for dry skin conditions.

Scientific evidence does not support reports that oats may help counteract nicotine addiction, but does support the effectiveness of oats' traditional uses as an antidepressant and cardiac tonic.

Doctors often prescribe an oatmeal pack or mask for fighting psoriasis; for reducing wrinkles it is much less expensive and often just as effective as commercial anti-aging preparations.

OLIVE. *Olea europea.* Olive oil is used widely in herbal medicine as a vehicle for binding other herbs and as a solvent for chemical components. Olive oil alone is also used externally as an emollient, a softener of ear wax, and a skin lubricant. It is used internally as a laxative, taken either orally or as an enema. An old folk remedy to avoid intoxication calls for taking olive oil by the spoonful prior to drinking. This use is backed by research showing that olive oil coats the stomach wall, inhibiting absorption of alcohol and promoting its excretion while enzymes break down the alcohol. Olive oil also raises blood sugar, giving a boost of energy much like that of sugar. A bark infusion is drunk to help eliminate worms, and is used as a wash for skin ulcers and sores.

ONION. *Allium cepa.* Raw onion (see illustration on page 21) is eaten to treat anemia, exhaustion, stomach gas, and bronchial problems. Decocted onion water is drunk as a tea to relieve sore throats and reduce coughs.

Onion is applied externally as a poultice to sores, bites, and burns. Roasted onion is poulticed to boils to draw them out. Onion also promotes healing of wounds and acts as an antibiotic, much like garlic. Some people eat onions to reduce blood sugar, hypertension, cholesterol, and inflammation. Onions are a rich source of vitamins B and C.

OREGANO. *Origanum vulgare* and other species. Known primarily as a pizza flavoring, this member of the mint family is effective in the treatment of upset stomach, vomiting, and diarrhea and as a digestive aid. There are some 40 herbs known as oregano, so identification may not always be precise.

An infusion of oregano is used to settle the stomach after a heavy meal or greasy foods have been eaten, and as a cold-fighting medicine. Some of the herbs sold as oregano are easily grown in the southern United States. It can be propagated from cuttings and grown from seeds.

Wild oregano may also be known as wild marjoram. In Mexico the dried flowers and leaves are brewed into an infusion taken to relieve PMS symptoms, regulate menstrual flow, and reduce cramps. A double-strength oregano tea is used to loosen intestinal parasites and expel them. Milder tea is used to loosen and expel phlegm and relieve bronchitis.

OSWEGO TEA. *Monarda didyma.* Another aromatic member of the mint family, this plant is named for one of the Indian tribes that used it to treat colds and sore throats and to clear sinuses. It is a perennial plant that spreads when established, flourishing best in moist places. It is grown by many to attract hummingbirds, butterflies, and bees and is sold as bee balm.

PAPAYA. *Carica papaya.* This tropical fruit has come to the United States from South and Central America. Eating the fruit is beneficial for problems of the digestive process, from improving appetite and metabolism to relieving indigestion. Papain, an enzyme obtained from papayas, is used in making meat tenderizers and pills that aid digestion. It is also used to soothe and heal damaged tissue. Raw papaya or its extracts can be applied to swollen tissue, sores and eruptions, and beestings for relief.

Mexican Indians taught Spanish colonists to put strips of papaya on wounds to heal and soothe them, and to rub the mashed papaya flesh on jellyfish stings to stop the burning. The juice of papaya is soothing to stomach ulcers and upset stomachs. In parts of Central America, a contraceptive tea for women is made by boiling the seeds. The leaves are brewed into a tea used to dispel worms; the tea made from the root acts as a diuretic.

PARSLEY. *Petroselinum crispum.* This herb came here from the eastern Mediterranean by way of England. Though it is usually considered a culinary herb, its medicinal usage goes back to ancient Rome and Greece, where it was taken as a food supplement to prevent gas and nausea. Today, it is used as a carminative and an aperient; also, some herbalists have found parsley, eaten fresh, to be a histamine blocker in its action, relieving itching and allergy symptoms. Since it is also a breath freshener, parsley is often served with meals containing a lot of garlic or other heavily scented spices and herbs.

Parsley herb, fresh or dried, can be placed in the nose to stop nosebleed. It is common for herbalists to brew parsley into a tea to treat and relieve kidney stones. A tea made from the crushed seeds is said to dry up a mother's milk after the baby is weaned; it is more commonly used to relieve menstrual cramps. Parsley-leaf poultices are applied to cuts, bites, and insect stings to relieve pain.

PASSIONFLOWER. *Passiflora incarnata* and other species. Passionflower, passion fruit, or maypop is often mislabeled as an aphrodisiac. The name refers not to human passion but to the Passion of Christ, a name given the beautiful purple flower by inspired Spanish priests, who called it *flos passionis.* It is said that a good Sunday-school teacher can tell the entire Crucifixion story from the flower parts and the leaves: the three-lobed leaf resembles the Roman spear that pierced Christ's side. The tendrils that help the vines to cling resemble the whips that beat Him. The five anthers represent the five wounds; the column of the ovary, the pillar of the cross; and the three styles, the three nails. The 10 sepals and petals represent the 10 apostles who remained faithful. The stamens represent the hammers that drove the nails through His hands and feet, and the calyx represents the glory, or nimbus, that surrounded Him. The wispy petals represent the crown of thorns, and the purple color of the blossom equates to the royal purple of the robe.

Passionflower leaves are used in commercial herbal sleep–inducing teas. They can be dried and stored for later use. It would seem unlikely that such an herb, used to induce sleep and reduce nervousness, could also be an aphrodisiac. I have successfully used about one tablespoon of crushed herb to a cup of boiling water to produce a tea for my wife when she could not sleep. It has also worked as an antispasmodic for upset stomach and seasickness.

The passionflower was formerly used as a nerve sedative to allay general restlessness and to relieve insomnia and certain types of convulsions and spasmodic disorders. Anodyne properties were also attributed to it, and it was used in the treatment of various neuralgias.

PIGWEED. *See* Plantain Herb.

PINE. *Pinus* species. The sap and the inner bark of many pine trees are used to make a syrup for relief of cough and sore throats. It also has expectorant qualities and so helps remove sputum and phlegm and relieve bronchial congestion. Pine is distilled into pine tar and turpentine, both of which have been used in veterinary medicine for the treatment of animals' sores and wounds and also in human medicine, used on the skin as an antiseptic. Pine needles steeped in boiling water provide a vitamin C–rich drink that is soothing to the throat. However, boiling the decoction over 20 minutes destroys the vitamin C and brings out an oil that acts as an expectorant.

A large quantity of fresh pine needles can be boiled and the water added to the bath for an invigorating and refreshing experience that helps stop itching caused by chiggers, sunburn, and other skin irritations.

PINEAPPLE. *Ananas comosus.* Most people do not think of pineapples as anything but a food, but they are grown commercially as a source of the meat-tenderizing chemical bromelain. Bromelain is also used in medical practice as a soft-tissue anti-inflammatory and in topical treatment of burns, wounds, and invasive injuries to the skin and soft tissue. Studies suggest that bromelain might be a natural nematicide (worm killer).

Unripe pineapples contain a violent purgative, and the juice and pulp could be used as a substitute for syrup of ipecac or other agents to empty the stomach of poisons or drug overdoses.

Pineapple juice works effectively as a diuretic.

PIPSISSEWA. *Chimaphila umbellata.* Pipsissewa is a Native American name for this plant referring to its use as an antilithic; it means "breaks into pieces." Its ability to dissolve kidney stones is questionable, but the tea made from the leaves does contain chemicals that soothe irritated kidney tissue, reduce inflammation and pain, and have antiseptic properties to fight infection. This native North American herb is found in moist woods. It is an evergreen with a white stripe adorning the leaves, giving rise to its other name, variegated wintergreen.

PITCHER PLANT. *Saracenia purpurea* and other species. In most places this endangered species is protected, so it should not be collected from the wild. Its leaves and roots can be brewed into a tea that calms the stomach and serves as both a diuretic and laxative, making it valuable in the treatment of obesity. Pitcher plants are carnivorous plants found in bogs across North America.

PLANTAIN BANANA. *Musa acuminata* or *M. paradisiaca.* Plantains are cooking bananas, so-called because generally they have very firm flesh and must be boiled, baked, or fried, or a combination of these, to be eaten. They are eaten as a vegetable when their skin is green or pale yellow and as a fruit when their skin has turned black. This is when they are at their sweetest as a fruit, but since most people think the color is a sign of having turned bad, we often see plantains at peak ripeness on the "Reduced for Quick Sale" rack. Plantains are most commonly misidentified as generic banana trees (not specifically plantains).

All bananas are Old World plants, coming from Asia, Africa, and the South Pacific, although they are now grown commercially in South and Central America, Hawaii, and the Caribbean. They are an important source of starch and potassium. A 100-gram (3½-ounce) portion of banana is 21 percent starch and contains roughly 380 milligrams of potassium. When ripe, bananas are very calorie-rich: 90 calories per 100 grams. Simply eating a banana has been known to completely alleviate the symptoms of patients who are having minor problems with breathing or circulation caused by an electrolytic imbalance. A family member who was very ill and appeared to be suffering from a severe flu attack was cured almost immediately by eating a banana. He had forgotten his supply of potassium pills, which were prescribed for an ongoing electrolyte imbalance. It is an excellent food for runners and others engaged in activities in which there is a great deal of sweating and fluid loss as well as caloric consumption. In the American tropics the plantain banana is referred to as a *platano*.

Plantain bananas are most commonly used in herbal medicine to cure or suppress viral wart growth. I once cured a friend who had warts across the knuckles of one hand by simply applying the inside portion of dried plantain peels to the affected area. The skins of noncooking bananas are also known to produce similar results. Apparently, an acid in the inner peel reduces the warts and also prevents growth of new ones. It may even kill the virus that causes the warts to grow. The thoroughly dried peels can be stored in an airtight container almost indefinitely and if need be can be moistened to make them easier to apply to the contours of the area where warts are found. When scanning other information sources, do not confuse plantain herb (see below) and plantain bananas.

PLANTAIN HERB. *Plantago* species. Plantain herb is one of my favorite herbs. It enjoys almost universal use in one form or another. Even today, many readers will be surprised to discover that they have in their medicine cabinets one of the greatest plant "pests," in the view of gardeners, greens keepers, and landowners. Psyllium hydrophilic mucaloid with dextrose, a generic bulk laxative, is a derivative of plantain herb. Although the generic form costs about one third as much as the brand-name equivalent, Metamucil, it is still relatively expensive and is a major rip-off for consumers. What that long generic name means is psyllium seed husks with sugar. Do you have any in your medicine chest? You can also find psyllium in these other commercial preparations: Konsyl, Effersyllium, Perdiem, Hydrocil, and others.

Psyllium comes from one of the plantain herbs, which are more commonly referred to as weeds. All of the plantain species are members of the genus *Plantago*; there are about 250 *Plantago* species worldwide. They were an Old World herb until the British conquered India and then this continent. Plantain herbs have such common names as pigweed (along with a dozen or so other plants), buckhorn, flea seed, and black, Spanish, or French psyllium. When plantain came to this country with the settlers, it spread so rapidly that several Native American tribes gave it a name that means "white man's foot!" Perhaps it came in animal droppings or was intentionally planted in some cases, but it was said that wherever the white man went this plant would spring up in his tracks. One of the common names for plantain, according to the well-known herbal medicine author Bradford Angier, is soldier's herb, so named because it was historically used to treat wounds in battle. Our own two most common varieties are *Plantago major*, or common plantain, and *P. lanceolata*, or narrow-leaf plantain. The true psyllium of the medical laxative trade is *Plantago ovata*, but the seed husks of other varieties are permitted by the FDA.

Only the husk from the seed is used in producing Metamucil and other laxatives. Mixed with water, the seed husks produce a mucilaginous mass that swells in the intestinal tract and pushes waste materials out slowly and safely. The seeds themselves are high in protein, but relatively difficult to digest when encased in the husk. The person who wishes to use plantain seeds as a protein source can either rub the seeds between the palms of the hands to remove the husks or use a hand grinder like a metate. The seeds can also be popped like popcorn; they are much smaller than popcorn kernels and are more easily digested. They can be roasted and then ground into flour or added to salads as a spice.

In hospital-based studies, psyllium seed has been shown to reduce hemorrhoids when applied topically, to reduce serum cholesterol when taken internally, and to raise blood sugar in certain diabetic patients. A tannin component has also been identified in the seeds, which gives them an astringent quality. Soaking the seeds in water yields a mucilage that is said to put life back in dry, abused hair.

Here is an interesting twist. We have already discussed the properties that make the seed husk and even the whole seed a bulk laxative. The green leaves and roots have a completely opposite effect. The tea that results from boiling the leaves has been shown to be astringent, and therefore it's a good antidiarrheal medicine. These same effects at one time gained plantain a place on the government's now barely mentioned GRAS, or "generally recognized as safe," list of herbs. It was reportedly good as an external poultice for tennis elbow and other similar sprains and pains. Folk medicine, through practical application, has shown that plantain leaves when "masticated" or otherwise crushed and applied to the site will relieve bee stings, hemorrhoids, poison ivy, and even the weeping blisters of sunburn.

Anecdotal evidence of plantain's healing abilities is supplied by a man who uses the alias of Robert Earthworm. He told me that he was once bitten on the toe by a rattlesnake and found himself confronting swelling, pain, and discoloration caused by the venom. He chewed plantain leaves and made a poultice, which he replaced frequently, and the swelling was resolved. I would never recommend this as a remedy against snakebite poisoning, but it's certainly worth a try if you are out in the middle of nowhere with no supplies and no chance of reaching assistance. For normal application, about one ounce of crushed, chopped plantain leaves is boiled in a pint or quart of water, but for reduction of hemorrhoids, the amount of leaves should be increased to about two ounces per cup of water.

While in the army, I tried a cold plantain-leaf tea as a wash on hemorrhoids, and it definitely stopped the itching and seemed to shrink them. I know of people who have used a chewed-plantain-leaf poultice to remove wood splinters or slivers. Certainly plantain leaves would be less toxic than a poultice of tobacco, which is sometimes recommended for splinters.

In one double-blind study it was shown that treating symptomatic hemorrhoids using the commercial preparation Vi-Siblin (which contains plantain) for three weeks produced an 84 percent relief rate. The placebo in the study produced a much smaller rate of symptomatic relief. The herbalist James A. Duke reports that Omaha Indians crushed the leaves and soaked them in oil and then applied the mixture to wounds to prevent scarring. He also tells us that the Penobscots of Maine used the roots in treating warts and cancer.

PLEURISY ROOT. *Asclepias tuberosus.* This member of the milkweed family is called butterfly root because its clear sap and orange flowers often attract butterflies. It doesn't transplant well but is easily grown from seed. The green part of the herb is toxic, but the dried root is made into a tea for treatment of pleurisy. It is especially popular in China for this and Chinese herbalists use it to relieve pain and swelling of the pleura, the sac that surrounds the lungs. It is also useful in treating smoker's cough and in reducing inflammation

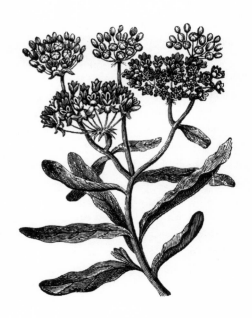

Pleurisy root

of the lungs following accidents or trauma that make breathing difficult.

POTATO. *Solanum tuberosum.* Although it originally came from South America, this staple vegetable (see illustration on page 20) is, ironically, called the Irish potato in this country and the Virginia potato in Ireland. It has been used in Native American and Mexican medicine for centuries; more recently, modern science has discovered in the potato a high level of chlorogenic acid, a substance believed to prevent cellular mutations that lead to cancer.

The raw, expressed juice can be drunk to relieve stomachache, diarrhea, and fluid retention. Some herbalists and native healers place slices of potato on the temples to cure headaches, and raw potato is mashed and applied as a poultice to treat puffiness of eyelids, cracked skin, sunburn, and insect bites.

POKEWEED. *Phytolacca americana.* Pokeweed should be excluded from the herbalist's medical repertoire. All parts of the plant are poisonous, with the exception of the unfolded leaves for a brief period in the spring. Perhaps for this reason, poke enjoys a reputation as a spring tonic, particularly in the South. (Spring tonics are traditionally used to cleanse the body, purify the blood and stimulate the appetite and, depending upon their ingredients, may also act as laxatives and nutritional supplements). Many field guides neglect to mention that foods called poke salad or sallet cannot be eaten raw but must be cooked in at least two changes of water.

Many Indian tribes used the dried roots as a vermifuge, taking minute doses, a little at a time, and waiting for the effect. This is not recommended, however, since the plant's substances work on the central nervous system and are therefore dangerous. Poke can be used to relieve the pain of arthritis, but because of the hazards related to poke use, trained herbalists, knowing their own limitations, use dried poke berries as pills for this purpose, not the leaves or roots. I once found the sixty-plus-year-old Dot Montgillion, an herbalist in West Virginia who dries the berries for her own use, up in a cherry tree picking fruit, her arthritic pains mitigated by poke berry treatment.

Native Americans used poke roots and berries to treat cancers and boils, and it is used in commercial cancer treatments today.

POMEGRANATE. *Punicum granatum.* Mentioned in the Bible many times, pomegranate comes to us from the Middle East but is now cultivated in many places. The pulp of the fruit is eaten as a food, but the rind is made into a tea that is an effective vermifuge as well as an astringent tea for treating diarrhea. The tea is also especially effective against tapeworms and other intestinal parasites: it causes them to relax their grip so that they can be expelled by a purgative.

PRICKLY ASH. *Zanthoxylum americanum.* The prickly ash is not related to the ash trees, but is a thorn-studded shrub belonging to the rue family. It is specifically known as the toothache tree because chewing its bitter bark relieves the pain of toothache.

PRICKLY PEAR. *Opuntia* species. This cactus family includes plants that vary from those that grow tall into hedge or bush form to some that become rambling, prostrate forms that stay flat, near the ground. The pads are sold as an exotic vegetable, available either cut up and canned (called *nopales*) in the Mexican food section of the market, or fresh, especially in areas with a large Hispanic population. The leaves, or pads, can be split open and applied to burns, sores, and wounds, much like aloe vera. When boiled, they yield a mucilage that is an excellent treatment for stomach ulcers, sore throats, and inflamed tonsils.

The fruits are sold as Indian pears, tunas, or cactus pears and are a better source of vitamin C than oranges or other citrus fruits. The Aztecs drank the juice and mixed it with egg yolks to treat burns.

PUFFBALL. *Lycoperodon* and *Calvatia* species. When these fungi shrivel up and dry they become a shell full of a fine brown powder— the spores. These spores are applied to a wound to stop bleeding.

PULSATILLA. *Anemone pulsatilla.* Known to some as pasque flowers or wind flowers, this herb was popular in Europe and Russia, where the entire herb was made into a liquid extract used to relieve nervous exhaustion, as a sedative for catarrh, and to relieve absence of menstruation caused by stress. Today it is available in liquid extracts and tablets and is used to treat blood pressure problems as well as spasms of the uterine wall and the stomach.

PUMPKIN *(Winter squash).* *Cucurbita pepo* and *C. maxima.* Native to tropical America, pumpkins now are cultivated around the world and are most commonly used as a food. Native Americans used the pulp to treat burns and the seeds as a kidney medicine or to ease the

tive substances can cause uterine contractions that result in miscarriage or premature birth. Rosemary tea is an effective carminative. The crushed leaves can be applied as a temporary relief for toothaches.

RUE. *Ruta graveolens.* Care should be exercised when using rue internally because it is a uterine stimulant and could lead to spontaneous abortion, and externally it may cause photodermatitis. This characteristic has been taken advantage of in darkening white spots on the skin known as leucodermas. Used cautiously as an infusion, rue is an effective antispasmodic and emmenagogue.

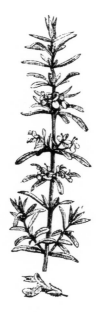

Rosemary

SAGE. *Salvia officinalis.* Some call sage a wonder herb and many herbalists recommend it be used alone rather than in any combination, which might weaken its strength. Sage dries up mucous secretions, and sage tea is used for such diverse purposes as ending lactation to facilitate weaning a baby, curing gum disease, and acting as a decongestant. Sage also works to slow perspiration, which can have positive or negative effects, depending on the situation.

Sage tea relieves headaches in many people and, with its anti-inflammatory properties, reduces fevers. Some people take sage tea as a natural cure for depression. Asthmatics smoke sage leaves for relief (like mullein, it relaxes the bronchi and reduces the "tickle" cough trigger), and some persons ingest sage to prevent an upset stomach when eating foods known to cause gastric distress.

Sage tea is used by some as a coffee substitute; weak sage tea is given to prevent or fight diarrhea. Used as a mouthwash, it not only reduces swollen gums but also fights the bacteria that cause gum disease. The tea is used externally as a wash for wounds to prevent infection.

ST. JOHN'S WORT. *Hypericum perforatum.* This herb, growing wild in North America, is used to heal wounds and fight viruses and acts as an astringent. Recent studies suggest that St. John's wort may be effective in AIDs treatment by helping to boost the immune system. In medieval Europe it was used to fight melancholia and other mental disorders. Native Americans diffused it for treating tuberculosis and other respiratory ailments. To treat sore throat, lung ailments, and urinary infections, make a tea of one tablespoon herb to a half pint of water. This has also been used in treating bedwetting.

St. John's oil is made by soaking the chopped herb in olive oil for a two-week period. This can be used for treating burns, bruises, and wounds and for the external treatment of soft-tissue injuries such as strains, sprains, and bruises.

Hypericin, an ingredient in St. John's wort, may cause skin burning in light-skinned photosensitive persons. For this reason, the FDA declared it unsafe in 1977, following blistering in cattle who had eaten large quantities. This has not stopped the FDA from allowing the same herb to be used in flavoring vermouth.

Because St. John's wort contains chemicals that act as monoamine oxidase inhibitors, which retard the breakdown of the neurotransmitters serotonin and neurepinephrine, it is good for treating depression, insomnia, and anxiety disorders.

SARSAPARILLA. *Smilax* species. These vines are unforgettable, once encountered. The small ones are called catbriers (because of their tiny claws) or green briers (because no matter how mature they get, the stems always stay green); the big ones are called "waita–minute–vines" by soldiers. The roots are used as alteratives and anti–inflammatory and antipruritic (anti–itch) agents as well as in the treatment of skin diseases. Chinese varieties are used by traditional healers there for treating rheumatism, dysentery, and syphilis. Sarsaparonin tablets have been shown to be effective in treating psoriasis.

When the root is boiled it produces a tea that is drunk to purify the blood, which in turn prevents skin eruptions and diseases. It also contains a substance called sarapogenin, which is similar to progesterone and may help with premenstrual bloating and fluid retention.

Sarsaparilla is an effective diuretic and reduces blood pressure, but taken in large quantities it may cause electrolyte imbalances—a problem encountered when using any effective diuretic. It has been officially used to treat syphilis in the United States and China and is suggested by some native healers and herbalists as a treatment in leprosy.

A leaf tea is used by experienced herbalists to counteract poisons in some cases. This tough, twining vine, a member of the lily family, may be collected in most regions of the United States. Although they have no medicinal value, the young tendrils are quite tasty and may be eaten raw or cooked (I add them to stir–fry recipes). In some species, the root can be boiled and will produce a tasty Jello-O–like substance when it cools.

SASSAFRAS. *Sassafras albidum.* Many turned away from sassafras tea a few years ago when it was listed as a carcinogen by the FDA. The controversy has been somewhat diminished by foreign studies that conclude it isn't as dangerous as many other substances ingested by Americans every day, including beer and mustard in packets. Sassafras is a very good diuretic and was used by Native Americans for reducing blood pressure, dissolving kidney stones, and as a blood tonic. The roots are used for making tea and root beer. The dried leaves are turned into the spice called file (FEE-lay) powder, a popular ingredient in Cajun cooking (as in "file gumbo").

One friend of mine used the tea to effectively bring down chronic high blood pressure without using the prescribed medicine so that the family doctor stopped the prescription. However, it is never recommended to stop using a prescribed medicine and substitute herbs for it without consulting your health-care practitioner.

SAW PALMETTO. *Serenoa repens.* The berries of this shrubby palm tree, also known as sabal palm, have been used traditionally to correct urinary tract disorders, impotency, BPH (benign prostatic hypertrophy), and reduced libido, and to increase fertility and lactation in women. While it has been shown to naturally increase breast size in some persons, in others it has been shown to increase adipose (fatty) tissue over the entire body. Saw palmetto berries are used as a diuretic, an expectorant, a mild sedative, and an appetite stimulant. They have also been used to reverse thyroid deficiency.

Saw palmetto is now available as a standardized product and is used to inhibit conversion of testosterone into DHT (dihydrotestosterone), an agent causing enlarged prostate.

SENNA. *Cassia marilandica.* This herb, which grows wild in the southern United States, is the source of the senna or cassia used in commercial laxative preparations. (A variety of species are found in other parts of the world.) Native Americans also used senna as a laxative and for treating fever. Senna is used in federal hospitals to treat constipated soldiers and veterans, despite the fact that the government is extremely conservative when it comes to herbal medicine.

SHEEP SORREL. *Rumex acetosella.* This wild herb has an easily recognized arrowhead-shaped leaf and is found growing throughout North America and Europe. High in vitamin C, it is used as a diuretic and to treat urinary tract and vitamin C–deficiency problems. It also acts as a laxative and antiseptic.

SKULLCAP. *Scutellaria laterifolia.* This member of the mint family grows in North America and on other continents. It has been called mad dog weed because of its use in treating rabies. Native Ameri-

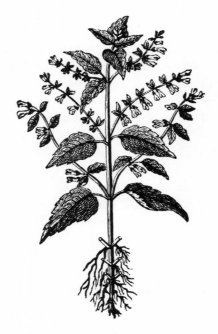

Skullcap

cans turned to it as a tranquilizer, digestive aid, and sedative. The herb is brewed into a tea that is currently recommended to treat nervous tension, anxiety, PMS, and the effects of drug and alcohol withdrawal.

SLIPPERY ELM. *Ulmus rubra.* Slippery elm is mentioned in early country doctor journals and in records of encounters with Native Americans who used it in treating sore throats, coughs and congestion, and wounds. Early throat lozenges were made from slippery elm bark and a modern version is still available in drug and health stores. The bark contains a large quantity of mucilage, which helps in soothing irritated mucous membranes and irritated stomach and bowel linings. The bitter decoction is sweetened with sugar and drunk for duodenal ulcers.

SOAPWORT. *Saponaria officinalis.* This important herb, which grows wild in Europe and the United States, is used medicinally to treat most skin diseases and eruptions. Also known as bouncing Bet, it is high in saponins (lather-producing substances) and when agitated in water produces an antibacterial lather that can be used as a soap substitute. In England it is used to produce a head on some beers. *See also* Bouncing Bet.

STRAWBERRY. *Fragaria* species. The strawberry plant (see illustration on page 23) needs no identification to most people, particularly herbalists. Though the fruit is the most commonly used portion, the leaves can be brewed into a tea that is very high in vitamin A. With its mildly astringent and diuretic properties, this tea is also useful in treating diarrhea and sore throats.

SUMA. *Pfafia paniculata.* One of the most highly regarded traditional herbs of South American healers, this plant is known as Brazilian ginseng, although it is really in the amaranth family. In Spanish it is known as *para todo,* which means "for everything," indicating its panacea effect. A true adaptogen, it is available now as a standardized product and is used as an anabolic, similar to steroids, analgesic and anti-inflammatory and to increase stress resistance. The root is harvested and various substances, including vitamins A, B1, B2, and E, are extracted from it in the form of a juice, distillation, or solution.

SWEET GUM. *Liquidambar styraciflua.* This giant tree, a member of the witch hazel family, is currently listed in the U.S. Pharmacopeia as a source of storax, an expectorant and antiseptic. It is native to North America and produces a gum or sap that has been used for chewing gum, to flavor Montezuma's smoking mixture (an Aztec blend of tobacco, sweet gum, and different available herbs) and as a skin medicine, ringworm treatment, and hemorrhoid cure.

TANSY. *Tanacetum vulgare.* This strong-smelling perennial is also known as bitter buttons because of its rather small, yellow flowers. Introduced from Europe, this herb has long been popular as an anthelminthic and emmenagogue. Scientific studies show it has some value as an antispasmodic, due to its ability to relax the stomach muscles. The leaves are infused and drunk as a bitter tonic. Its most popular use today may be topically as an insect repellant.

TARRAGON. *Artemesia dracunculus.* Known best as a culinary herb, tarragon is also used in medicine as a diuretic and an appetite stimulant. When taken as an infusion, it is also good for alleviating the pain of arthritis. The leaves can be chewed to relieve the pain of toothache or tooth removal as tarragon numbs the mouth and throat. It contains the oil, eugenol, which is used in some toothache drops.

THYME. *Thymus vulgaris.* Though an essential flavoring for soups and stews and an ingredient in the culinary herb mixture, bouquet garni, thyme is also used medicinally. Thyme tea is used to relieve spasms and coughing, to calm whooping cough, and as an antispasmodic. Strong thyme decoctions are thought to be capable of inducing abortion, but a weaker tea is used to elininate phlegm and reduce postnasal drip. Strangely, cold thyme tea is used to treat headaches while hot thyme tea is used to induce sleep and to help overcome shortness of breath. Hot thyme infusion is also good for relieving stomach cramps and diarrhea. Externally, thyme poultices or washes made from infusions can be effective against wounds and cuts as an antiseptic.

TOADFLAX. *Linaria vulgaris.* Known to some as butter and eggs because of its flowers' color and appearance, this plant is used in tea form as a mouthwash to fight sores and infections, and as a liver

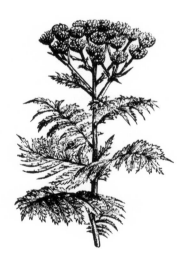

Tansy

stimulant. The flowering stems are also brewed into a tea to stimulate a sluggish liver and increase the production of bile.

TRAGACANTH. *Astragalus gummifer.* More commonly referred to as astragalus (not to be confused with astragalus membranaceus) or tragacanth gum, it is used by herbalists to bind other herbs together and is available in many herb shops and from suppliers. The gum is the dried sap exudate of a tree that grows in the Middle East, especially Turkey. Recent studies show that tragacanth itself may have some immune system–stimulating effects, but mostly it is known for its use in thickening emulsions, syrups, and other preparations and in making pills.

TURMERIC. *Curcuma longa.* One of the main ingredients in curry powder, turmeric has also been used historically as a gallbladder tonic and as a treatment for hepatitis and liver disease, as well as for bile duct problems. It is also used to treat arthritis, prevent cancer, and help combat obesity. Turmeric contains chemicals that lower blood cholesterol, reduce blood pressure, and metabolize fats. When the adrenal glands are working properly, turmeric also exhibits a nonsteroidal anti–inflammatory effect. The rhizome is the part of the plant used and it is now sold in standardized botanical preparation as 100 mg capsules to be taken with meals to protect against cancer, lower cholesterol, and treat arthritis. Turmeric also exhibits antifungal and antibacterial activities, which may help explain its ability to retard spoilage in meats. Because it lowers cho-

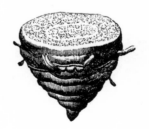

Turmeric

lesterol, turmeric is being used to prevent heart disease in some patients.

Powdered turmeric can be applied externally to wounds to prevent infection. Some hunters use this form as first aid for hunting dogs while on trips far from home.

An infusion made from about one teaspoon of turmeric in a cup of warm milk makes a relaxing, healthy bedtime drink. Larger amounts become somewhat bitter.

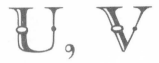

U, V

VALERIAN. *Valeriana officinalis.* Native to Europe, valerian has become naturalized in the United States and may be found growing wild as well as cultivated. The root is the part used, and valerian's strong, unique smell makes it easy to recognize. This is "nature's Valium": historically it has been used as a sedative and tranquilizer to treat insomnia, nervous tension, palpitations of the heart, epilepsy, children's behavioral disorders, and anxiety. Some sources say that large amounts can cause headaches, grogginess, and nausea, and other accounts warn of an addiction potential, though this is undocumented. The root is collected in the spring and dried; the roots can be used right away or stored for later use. A dose of two teaspoonsful of powdered root is steeped in a cup of water for 15 minutes and drunk before bedtime to promote a good night's sleep. It is usually sweetened to

twigs, and bark are soaked in water or alcohol and distillation removes the active principle, which is used as a topical cooling agent and to relieve the itching of poison ivy and the pains of sprains and strains, sunburn, and insect bites. Herbalists make a poultice of the leaves for the same purposes. Commercially available witch hazel products are not intended for internal use, but infusions from fresh or dried leaves have been cautiously used for treatment of internal hemorrhage and to relieve excessive menstrual flow. A cold wash is used externally to reduce and relieve piles.

WORMWOOD. *Artemesia absinthium.* Wormwood was once recommended by herbalists for the treatment of intestinal parasites, hence the name. The FDA has declared it unsafe, and a popular Middle Eastern narcotic alcoholic beverage distilled from wormwood, called absinthe, is banned from the United States—even though tiny amounts of wormwood are used to flavor vermouth. In large doses, wormwood causes insomnia and nightmares and is reputed to cause mental illness when used regularly.

X, Y, Z

YARROW. *Achillea millefolium*. People who bleed easily when shaving would do well to learn to identify this plant. It gets its scientific name from the Greek hero Achilles and accounts tell us that his soldiers were saved from bleeding to death when the medical people with his troops stuffed this plant into the men's arrow and spear wounds, stanching the flow of blood. *Millefolium* means "thousand-leaf" and refers to the fernlike appearance of the leaves, which some say resembles thousands of small leaves. Yarrow can be used to stop a bloody nose, known as epistaxis by physicians. Wound-wort and nosebleed are two of the common names of yarrow. Yarrow tea, made from one ounce of herb to a pint of water, has been used to treat bleeding ulcers and fevers. The antipyretic properties of yarrow are due to its salicylic acid. Yarrow has been used as a hypotensive by some to lower blood pressure.

Blood Pressure–Lowering Tea

1 ounce dried yarrow
1 pint water
1 ounce ground sassafras root

Boil water and steep herbs, covered, until tea is cool enough to drink.

This tea is also used in the treatment of diarrhea, colds, and rheumatism.

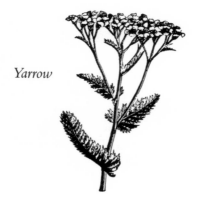

Yarrow

Sore Throat Gargle

1 teaspoon yarrow
1 teaspoon sage
1 teaspoon plantain
1 teaspoon mullein leaf or root

All the herbs should be dried. Mix together and pour one quart of boiling water over the herbs. Steep 15 minutes, sweeten with honey if desired, and gargle as needed when cool. Refrigerate unused portion.

The sage will help assuage the headache that accompanies sore throat and the other herbs will promote healing.

YELLOW BEDSTRAW. *Gallium verum.* According to legend, this is the plant that the Blessed Mary prepared the Christ child's manger with, but it is probably far better known as the source of a cheese-curdling agent and two dyes, red from the roots and yellow from the flowers. We find it in botanical shampoos for blondes. Medicinally we find it used as a diuretic and in the treatment of epilepsy. Its most easily verifiable use, due to its blood-clotting properties, is as a styptic.

YELLOW FLAG. *Iris pseudoacorus.* Common in much of the southeastern United States, this herb should not be taken internally, although it was once used as a diuretic and emetic. It was widely used in Europe and was brought to America during colonization. In France, a nineteenth-century chemist discovered that the roasted seeds can be made into a brew that tastes similar to coffee. A lotion or salve made from the roots is sometimes recommended for sores on the skin, breaks in the sole of the foot, and rough, chapped hands.

YELLOW JESSAMINE. *Gelsemium sempervivens.* Mentioned here as an herb to avoid because of its effect on the central nervous system as a depressant, yellow jessamine is more commonly mentioned in poison-plant books than medicinal herbals. Also known as Carolina jasmine or yellow jasmine, this evergreen vine sports a poison that has been compared to that of the deadly hemlock with which Socrates was forced to end his own life. Some older references will recommend this plant in treating pain, fever, and stomach spasms, but it is an extremely dangerous plant and should be avoided entirely.

YELLOW ROOT. *Xanthorhiza simplicissima.* Herbalists believe that excessive doses of this herb may be harmful. Used by Native Americans and popular in Appalachia since Daniel Boone's day, it's most commonly taken as a bitter tonic, stimulating the appetite and remedying stomach upset. The outer bark of the yellow root is where the active principles are, but often the whole root is brewed into a tea. This tea can be used as a mouthwash for sores and cankers. Chewing the root helps cleanse the mouth and sharpens the sense of taste. Since gathering it is not economical enough to warrant the research given a new drug, it is currently not very popular with pharmacists.

YERBA SANTA. *Eriodictyon californicum.* The leaves of this evergreen shrub are prepared into tea that is an expectorant and is used to treat bronchitis and asthma, and because of its aromatic flavor and taste is used to mask the taste of quinine and other bitter drugs.

YEW. *Taxus baccata* and *T. cuspidata.* Despite its recent celebrity as a cancer-treating-drug source, almost the entire yew plant is toxic and several human deaths have been recorded. The average herbalist is unable to extract the anticancer principles and should not attempt use of this herb. The Celts were said to tip their arrows with sap from yew trees because it was a nerve poison and would paralyze their enemies.

YOHIMBE. *Pausinystalia yohimbe.* For centuries the bark of yohimbe has been used in African medicine as a sexual stimulant, and it was brought to this country for its aphrodisiac qualities and as a hallucinogen. Science is investigating it as a treatment for organic impotence, but the average consumer would do well to avoid it. High dosages can lead to depression. Yohimbe bark bought from street sources may or may not be the real thing, and the active ingredient in store purchases is difficult to monitor. Too much yohimbe can lead to hypotension and central nervous system stimulation followed by paralysis.

ZEA MAYS. *See* Cornsilk.

Appendix A

Ailments

Please note that the listings under "Herb" refer only to the main entries in this book. You will have to read the entire entry to find out exactly what part of the herb is used to treat the condition you wish to alleviate. This is very important, as the different parts of an herb can serve different purposes. For instance, dried rhubarb roots are a powerful antidiarrhea medicine, while rhubarb leaf stalks act as a laxative. Rhubarb leaves themselves, however, are poisonous. Make sure you read the entry completely before considering any herbal preparations.

CONDITION	HERB
Acne	*bouncing Bet, elm, garlic, horsetail, soapwort*
Alcohol withdrawal symptoms	*alfalfa, angelica, kudzu, skullcap, valerian*

Alcohol tremors	*cayenne*
Allergy symptoms and allergic reactions	*echinacea, jujube, kombucha, nettle, parsley*
Alzheimer's disease	*ginkgo, marigold*
Amenorrhea (irregular menstruation)	*arbor vitae, chaste berry, chaste tree, ephedra, fennel, fenugreek, gentian, horehound, juniper, lovage, mint, pulsatilla, rosemary, rue, tansy, vanilla*
Anemia	*amaranth, blue cohosh, dong quai, nettle, onion, watercress*
Angina	*willow*
Anxiety and tension	*chamomile, black cohosh, black walnut, catnip, kava kava, lady's slipper, lemongrass, linden, mistletoe, passionflower, pulsatilla, St. John's wort, skullcap, valerian*

Appendix A

Appetite, to control

*artichoke, chickweed,
dandelion, vervain*

Appetite, to stimulate

*beech, devil's claw, fennel,
feverbush, gentian, ginger,
ginkgo, ginseng, hops,
mugwort, papaya, saw
palmetto, tarragon, yellow root*

Arthritis and rheumatism

*aloe vera, angelica, barley,
birch, bladderwrack, bloodroot,
boneset, cayenne, devil's claw,
devil's club, dogwood, dyer's
weed, echinacea, evening
primrose, feverfew, gentian,
goldenseal, hyssop, Joe-Pye-
weed, juniper, kalmia, luffa,
mustard, nettle, pokeweed,
rosemary, sarsaparilla, suma,
tarragon, turmeric, vervain,
violet, wild yam, willow,
wintergreen*

Asthma

*bamboo, chamomile, devil's
dung, echinacea, eucalyptus,
feverfew, garlic, ginkgo, kola
nut, marigold, mullein, sage,
yerba santa*

Appendix A

Athlete's foot	*black walnut*
Back pain	*gentian, hydrangea, luffa, willow*
Bedwetting	*mullein, St. John's wort*
Bladder and kidney infections	*cornsilk, cranberry, dodder, horsetail, Irish moss, kinnikinnick, mallow, pumpkin*
Bleeding gums	*amaranth, bayberry, bilberry, echinacea, watercress*
Bleeding, external	*horsetail, puffball, yarrow, yellow bedstraw*
Bleeding, internal	*dead nettle, nettle, witch hazel*
Bloating, abdominal	*celery seed, dandelion, marigold, mate, sarsaparilla, watercress*

Boils and abscesses

*burdock, echinacea, elm,
evening primrose, fenugreek,
fig, goldenseal, horsetail,
indigo, Joe-Pye-weed,
marijuana, olive, onion,
soapwort*

Bone fractures

comfrey

Bronchitis

*cacao, coltsfoot, elecampane,
ephedra, eucalyptus, garlic,
horehound, hyssop, Irish moss,
juniper, luffa, marijuana,
mint, mullein, mustard,
onion, oregano, pine,
watercress, yerba santa*

Bruises

*arnica, hyssop, jewelweed,
St. John's wort*

Burns

*aloe vera, borage, balsam fir,
bamboo, beech, comfrey, flax,
garlic, jewelweed, Joe-Pye-
weed, jojoba, mallow,
marigold, oak, oats, onion,
pineapple, prickly pear,
pumpkin, St. John's wort*

Caffeine withdrawal

beech, cacao, cleavers, dandelion, kola nut, sage

Calluses

marigold

Cancer prevention

acerola, alum root, blessed thistle, bloodroot, broccoli, devil's dung, echinacea, evening primrose, garlic, indigo (wild), licorice, marijuana, marjoram, mayapple, pokeweed, pumpkin, red clover, turmeric

Canker sores

acacia gum, balsam fir, blackberry, sage, toadflax, yellow root

Cardiac arrythmias

ginkgo, night-blooming cereus

Cellulite

kombucha

Chapped lips

jojoba

Chilblains

garlic, ginkgo, Jew's ear

Childbirth
See Labor pain

Cholesterol, high

artichoke, flax, garlic, ginger, onion, turmeric

Circulatory problems

cayenne, dong quai, ginger, horseradish, luffa, marigold, mugwort, rosemary

Cirrhosis of the liver

licorice

Colds and flu

acacia gum, acerola, alder, boneset, cacao, catnip, echinacea, ephedra, garlic, ginger, goldenrod, marigold, mustard, oregano, Oswego tea, red clover

Cold sores
See also Herpes

ash, balm, camphor, cayenne, comfrey, lavender, luffa

Colic

angelica, catnip, chamomile, fennel, lovage, wild yam

Appendix A

Congestion, chest

devil's dung, eucalyptus, ginger, ground ivy, horehound, hyssop, ipecac, jewelweed, juniper, licorice, luffa, mint, mustard, oregano, pine, red clover, saw palmetto, slippery elm, sweet gum, thyme, violet

Congestion, head and nose

ephedra, ginger, luffa, magnolia, mint, Oswego tea, red clover, sage

Conjunctivitis (pinkeye)

barberry

Constipation, in adults

aloe vera, apples, ash, asparagus, boneset, broom, cascara sagrada, castor oil, cayenne, culver's root, cumin, dodder, dogwood, dyer's weed, elder, feverfew, flax, ginseng, kola nut, lavender, marsh marigold, olive, parsley, pitcher plant, plantain herb, rhubarb, rose hips, sage, senna, sheep sorrel, walnut

Constipation, in children

elder

Appendix A

Corns

fig

Coughs

acacia, alder, anise, bamboo, bayberry, cayenne (capsicum), coltsfoot, elecampane, fig, garlic, ginger, goldenrod, gum, horehound, hyssop, ipecac, Irish moss, luffa, marigold, marijuana, marshmallow, marsh marigold, onion, pine, slippery elm, thyme, violet

Cuts, abrasions, and sores

balsam fir, bayberry, bladderwrack, borage, bouncing Bet, burdock, chickweed, comfrey, coriander, garlic, hyssop, indigo, mallow, onion, papaya, parsley, pineapple, prickly pear, sage, St. John's wort, thyme, turmeric, virgin's bower, walnut, yellow flag

Cystitis
See Urinary tract infections
and cystitis

Dandruff

eucalyptus, garlic, soapwort

Appendix A

Dehydration

kaolin

Depression

balmony, basil, borage, cloves, oats, St. John's wort

Diabetes

alfalfa, celery seed, devil's club, fenugreek, ginseng, Jerusalem artichoke, watercress

Diaper rash

burdock, comfrey, marigold, plantain herb

Diarrhea and dysentery

acacia gum, agrimony, alum root, amaranth, anise, apples, ash, bael, balsam fir, barberry, beech, blackberry, black walnut, dead nettle, elecampane, garlic, indigo (wild), kaolin, knotweed, marigold, mesquite, nutmeg, oak, oregano, pomegranate, potato, raspberry, rhubarb, sage, sarsaparilla, strawberry, thyme, water lily, wintergreen

Drug overdose

birch, boneset, garlic, ipecac, kelp, milk thistle, pineapple

Appendix A

Drug withdrawal symptoms	*skullcap*
Dry, chapped skin	*bladderwrack, eucalyptus, fenugreek, flax, jojoba, oats, olive, potato, violet, yellow flag*
Earache	*garlic, licorice, mullein*
Eczema	*burdock, chickweed, evening primrose, nettle, red clover, walnut*
Edema	*butcher's broom, devil's claw, elm*
Electrolyte imbalance	*barley, kelp, plantain banana*
Epilepsy	*lady's slipper, valerian, yellow bedstraw*
Exhaustion *See also* Lethargy	*bayberry, dong quai, ginger, ginseng, guarana, kola nut, mate, onion*

Appendix A

Eye irritation	*flax, goldenseal, horseradish, mesquite*
Eye problems (myopia, night blindness, etc.)	*bilberry, goldenseal*
Eye puffiness	*maple, potato*
Eye strain	*barley, bilberry, mesquite*
Fainting	*basil, horseradish*
Fever	*alder, ash, balm, blackberry, blessed thistle, boneset, borage, dogwood, echinacea, feverbush, feverfew, horehound, Joe-Pye-weed, lemongrass, luffa, rosemary sage, St. John's wort, senna, vervain, willow, yarrow*
Flatulence	*anise, calamus, fennel, fenugreek, ginger, goldenrod, lovage*

Flu
See colds and flu

Fluid retention

artichoke, asparagus, celery
seed, cornsilk, dandelion,
dyer's weed, echinacea, elder,
elm, fennel, goldenseal,
juniper, knapweed, kola nut,
lovage, marjoram, nettle,
papaya, pineapple, pitcher
plant, potato, rose hips,
sarsaparilla, sassafras, saw
palmetto, sheep sorrel,
strawberry, tarragon, vervain

Food poisoning

rosemary

Fungal skin infections

adder's tongue, aloe vera, black
walnut, chickweed, coriander,
echinacea, evening primrose,
fenugreek, goldenseal,
marigold, sarsaparilla,
soapwort, sweet gum, virgin's
bower, walnut

Gallbladder disorders

turmeric

Gastritis

angelica, balm, balmony, caraway, cinnamon, cumin, fenugreek, garlic, gentian, goldenrod, lemongrass, licorice, mallow, marigold, mint, onion, parsley, slippery elm

Gingivitis

sage

Glaucoma

marijuana

Goiter

kelp

Gout

devil's claw, dyer's weed, nettle, violet, willow

Gum disease
See Gingivitis

Hair loss

horsetail, jojoba, vervain

Halitosis

angelica, dill, fennel, lovage, parsley

Hay fever

echinacea, ground ivy, nettle

Headaches

aspirin, cayenne, fennel, feverfew, guarana, kola nut, lavender, magnolia, potato, pumpkin, rosemary, sage, skullcap, thyme, vervain, willow

Head injury

ginkgo

Heartburn
See Indigestion

Heart disease and heart problems

blessed thistle, dandelion, ephedra, garlic, ginkgo, hawthorn, magnolia, nettle, turmeric

Heat rash

marigold

Hemorrhoids (piles)

alder, aloe vera, butcher's broom, elder, ground ivy, indigo, luffa, mallow, mullein, nettle, oak, plantain herb, sweet gum, witch hazel

Hepatitis

garlic, licorice, turmeric

Herpes, genital
See also Cold sores

cayenne, comfrey, luffa, walnut

Hives

*evening primrose, fenugreek,
jewelweed*

Hyperactivity, in children

evening primrose, valerian

Hypertension (high blood
pressure)

*astragalus, barberry, black
cohosh, celery seed, dandelion,
dill, evening primrose,
feverfew, garlic, hawthorn,
jujube, mistletoe, nettle,
onion, pulsatilla, sassafras,
turmeric, yarrow*

Hypotension (low blood
pressure)

motherwort, rosemary

Hypoxia

ginkgo

Immune system, weak

*astragalus, barberry, boneset,
devil's claw, echinacea,*

ginseng, St. John's wort,
tragacanth

Impotence

cayenne, ginkgo, saw palmetto,
yohimbe

Incontinence

cranberry juice, kinnikinnick,
pumpkin

Indigestion and heartburn

artichoke, cacao, calamus,
caraway, cayenne, coriander,
culver's root, dandelion, devil's
claw, dill, fennel, feverfew,
gentian, goldenrod, hops,
horehound, indigo,
lemongrass, mint, nutmeg,
oregano, papaya, rosemary,
skullcap, vanilla

Insect bites and stings

aloe vera, comfrey, garlic,
indigo, jewelweed, mallow,
oak, oats, onion, papaya,
parsley, potato, witch hazel

Insect repellant

arbor vitae, black cohosh,
chamomile, garlic, mint, tansy

Appendix A

Insomnia (adults)	*chamomile, chaste berry, chaste tree, ginseng, hops, kava kava, lavender, linden, mint, passionflower, St. John's wort, thyme, turmeric, valerian*
Insomnia (children)	*chamomile, lavender*
Intestinal parasites	*black walnut, kamala, neem, oregano, pomegranate, pumpkin, tansy*
Iodine deficiency	*bladderwrack*
Irritable bowel syndrome and colitis	*barley, chamomile, hops, mesquite, slippery elm, wild yam*
Ischemia	*ginkgo*
Itchy skin	*kalmia, oak, oats, parsley, pine*

Appendix A

Kidney stones

hydrangea, knotweed, pipsissewa, sassafras

Labor pain

black cohosh, blue cohosh, life root, mugwort, raspberry

Leprosy

sarsaparilla

Lethargy

bayberry, dong quai, ginger, ginseng, guarana, kola nut, mate

Lice

delphinium, indigo, walnut

Liver disorders

artichoke, balmony, blessed thistle, cascara sagrada, dandelion, devil's claw, kombucha, licorice, milk thistle, toadflax, turmeric

Malaria

neem

Memory loss

ginkgo, marigold, rosemary

Menopausal syndrome	*chaste berry, chaste tree, dong quai, fennel, motherwort, mugwort*
Menstrual cycle, irregular *See also* Amenorrhea	*blue cohosh, chaste berry, chaste tree, fennel, fenugreek, gentian, horehound, juniper, lovage, mint, motherwort, oregano, pulsatilla, rosemary, rue, tansy*
Menstrual flow, excessive	*agrimony, blackberry, marigold, nettle, witch hazel*
Menstrual pain	*angelica, black cohosh, blue cohosh, butcher's broom, caraway, chaste berry, chaste tree, dong quai, feverfew, lavender, milk thistle, mugwort, oregano, parsley, pulsatilla, willow*
Morning sickness	*chamomile, ginger, mint, raspberry*
Motion sickness	*ginger, mint, passionflower*

Muscle cramps

alder, chamomile, wild yam

Muscle soreness or stiffness

arnica, birch, camphor, ginger, mint, willow

Nausea and vomiting

alum root, amaranth, anise, bael, caraway, cardamom, cloves, elecampane, fennel, gentian, ginger, lavender, marigold, marjoram, mint, nutmeg, oregano

Neuralgia

cayenne, lady's slipper, lavender, lemongrass, passionflower, St. John's wort

Nicotine withdrawal

cardinal flower, marigold, oats

Nosebleed

garlic, knotweed, nettle, parsley, yarrow

Obesity

kelp, pitcher plant, turmeric

Panic attack

black cohosh, black walnut, lady's slipper

Appendix A

Phlebitis   *bilberry*

Piles
See Hemorrhoids

Pinkeye
See Conjuncivitis

Pneumonia   *garlic, mint*

Poison, ingested   *birch, boneset, garlic, ipecac,*
                                            kelp, milk thistle, sarsaparilla,
                                            violet

Poison ivy and poison oak   *beech, bouncing Bet,*
                                            jewelweed, oak, oats, plantain
                                            herb, witch hazel

Pleurisy   *pleurisy root*

Premenstrual syndrome   *black cohosh, chaste berry,*
(PMS)   *chaste tree, dandelion, dong*
                                            quai, evening primrose,
                                            guarana, mate, oregano,
                                            sarsaparilla, skullcap, valerian

Appendix A

Prostate problems	cornsilk, horsetail, mallow, nettle, pygeum, saw palmetto
Psoriasis	bouncing Bet, cleavers, fig, oats, red clover, sarsaparilla, walnut, yellow flag
Rabies	skullcap
Respiratory problems	ground ivy, hyssop, mint, pleurisy root, St. John's wort
Ringworm	black walnut, sweet gum, walnut
Runny nose	thyme
Scabies	kalmia
Skin rashes	fenugreek, horsetail, jewelweed, Joe-Pye-weed, kalmia, luffa, marigold, oak, oats, pine, sweet gum

Sleep disorders

feverfew, guarana, kava kava, lavender, linden, marijuana, mint, passionflower, valerian

Smoker's cough

pleurisy root

Snakebite

echinacea, plantain herb

Sore throat

alum root, barberry, barley, bay berry, bladderwrack, bloodroot, borage, echinacea, elecampane, elm, fenugreek, fig, horehound, horseradish, Jerusalem artichoke, Jew's ear, linden, mallow, marjoram, marshamallow, oak, onion, Oswego tea, pine, prickly pear, St. John's wort, slippery elm, strawberry, tarragon, yarrow

Splinters

marijuana, plantain herb

Sprains and strains

alder, amaranth, arnica, birch, camphor, comfrey, kalmia, plantain herb, wintergreen, witch hazel

Staph infections

licorice

Stomach cramps

jalap, lavender, lovage, marjoram, motherwort, passionflower, pulsatilla, rue, thyme, vanilla

Stomach upset, adults

beech, black cohosh, caraway, cardamom, cascara sagrada, cinnamon, feverfew, licorice, luffa, marjoram, mint, oregano, papaya, pitcher plant, potato, slippery elm, vervain, yellow root

Stomach upset, children

chamomile

Strep throat

licorice, mallow, tarragon

Stress and nervous tension

balm, catnip, chamomile, ginseng, hops, kava kava, kola nut, lavender, lemongrass, passionflower, skullcap, suma, turmeric, valerian

Appendix A

Sunburn

aloe vera, jewelweed, jojoba, mallow, marigold, oats, pine, plantain herb, potato, prickly pear, witch hazel

Swollen glands and tonsils

mallow, marjoram, prickly pear

Syphilis

sarsaparilla

Tapeworm

black walnut, kamala, male fern, neem, olive, papaya, pomegranate, pumpkin, tansy

Teething pain, in children

chamomile, mallow, marshmallow

Testicles, swollen

luffa

Thyroid problems

saw palmetto

Toothaches, adult

alder, amaranth, catnip, cinnamon, cloves, garlic, mallow, marjoram, prickly ash, rosemary, tarragon, vervain, willow

Tonsillitis

echinacea, indigo (wild), Jew's ear, mallow, prickly pear

Tuberculosis

echinacea, lady's slipper, licorice, St. John's wort

Tumor

barberry

Ulcer, stomach

alder, angelica, bayberry, garlic, ginseng, goldenseal, horsetail, jujube, licorice, marigold, nettle, papaya, prickly pear, slippery elm, yarrow

Urinary tract infections and cystitis

cornsilk, cranberry, horsetail, hydrangea, Irish moss, kinnikinnick, licorice, St. John's wort, saw palmetto, sheep sorrel, vervain, willow

Urination, difficult

arbor vitae, artichoke, asparagus, burdock, cornsilk, horseradish, horsetail, hydrangea, kola nut, lovage, marjoram, nettle, papaya, pitcher plant, pygeum, sarsaparilla, sassafras, saw palmetto, sheep sorrel, tarragon, yellow bedstraw

Vaginal infections

comfrey

Vaginal itching

alder

Varicose veins

bilberry, butcher's broom, milk thistle

Vitamin A deficiency

broccoli, strawberry

Vitamin C deficiency

acerola, amaranth, broccoli, cleavers, cranberry, garlic, ground ivy, mate, onion, pine, prickly pear, rose hips, sheep sorrel, watercress

Warts

bloodroot, fig, marsh marigold, plantain banana, plantain herb

Whooping cough

coltsfoot, garlic, thyme

Yeast infection

dandelion, echinacea, licorice, oak

Appendix B

Resources

To make the most use of the country doctor's legacy of herbal folk medicine, it is important to use all of the resources that are available. In virtually every county in the nation, the local government's agriculture extension agents should know who is the expert on herbs from both a cultural point of view and a technical usage standpoint, whether that use be medicinal or culinary. If there are traditional healers where you live—Native American, African American, Asian American, or some other ethnicity—get to know them and, true to their calling, they will share their experience with you. Keep in mind, however, that acquiring this knowledge may be a slow and painstaking process.

Visit botanical gardens and museums that specialize in Native American or other cultural heritages and in herbs. In Bailey, North Carolina, a small town known for its bluebird houses built by Jack Finch, is the Museum of the Country Doctor, which is visited by the curious public, as well as by medical students, researchers, and herbalists from around the world.

But before traveling anywhere, first use your local resources. Look in the Yellow Pages of the phone book for any references to herbs, herbalists, or healers. Check them out carefully. Some so-called herbalists are only trained to sell the products they represent, while others may be a true fountain of knowledge. In Dayton, Ohio, herbal medicine classes have been taught at the hospital. At other locations they have been taught through community colleges or universities.

Join the Club

Virtually every state has at least one herb society. You can also join national groups that meet your needs.

The International Herb Association, formerly known as the International Herb Growers & Marketing Association (HGMA), 1202 Allenson Road, Mundelein, IL 60060, is the major commercial herb association in the country, but members come from all branches of the herb business and have many different interests. Their annual meeting is the best place to meet other herb professionals.

You can also join the American Herb Association, P.O. Box 1673, Nevada City, CA 95999, to learn more about the focus on herbal medicine.

Members of the Herb Research Foundation help support research into the reality of using herbs safely and effectively as medicines. Their address is 1007 Pearl Street, Suite 200, Boulder, CO 80302.

Professional herbalists will want to consider joining the American Herbalists Guild, P.O. Box 1683, Soquel, CA 95073, to work—and network—with other professionals.

Get Connected

There are a number of national publications that connect herbalists in a networking system to support commerce in herbs, research, and common interests.

The American Botanical Council and the Herb Research Foundation at P.O. Box 201660, Austin, TX 78720, is a great choice for those who want to seriously learn about herb research. Their magazine, *HerbalGram*, is the source of up-to-date information.

The Herbal Connection, P.O. Box 245, Silver Spring, PA 17575-0245 is a publication of the Herb Growing & Marketing Network and meets the needs of many herb growers, crafters, researchers, and consumers. The Herbal Green Pages, which are published once a year, are the equivalent of the Yellow Pages for herbalists.

You can find other herbal magazines and publications in your local bookstore or library.

Go High Tech

So far, only one herbal magazine is currently online, though others are sure to follow. Wouldn't the country doctor be amazed? *Alternative Medicine Digest* is, at this writing, the only full-length magazine on the Internet devoted solely to alternative health. Their address on the World Wide Web is http://www.alternativemedicine.com. Their regular address is Future Medicine Publishing, P.O. Box K, Milton, WA 98354-9902.

A couple of herbal medicine programs are now available on CD-ROM from Hopkins Technology, 421 Hazel Lane, Hopkins, MN 55343-7116. *The Herbalist*, a CD program by David L. Hoffman, covers basic principles, human systems, and herb actions and boasts an extensive *materia medica*, or plant listing. *Traditional Chinese Medicine and Pharmacology* covers basic principles, clinical experiences, herbal formulas and medicinal herb groups, as well as a *materia medica* of Chinese herb usage. Both CD-ROMs are available for Windows or Macintosh.

Appendix B

Go Back to School at Home

There are now a number of correspondence courses on the market devoted to the field of herbal medicine. My favorite is undoubtedly the Science and Art of Herbology course offered by Rosemary Gladstar through her school, SAGE, at P.O. Box 420, East Barre, VT 05649. Rosemary and I have been friends for years, I admit, ever since she ran the California School of Herbal Studies. But her course is more of an extension course than a correspondence course, because you will be required to grow some herbs, do some experiments and hands-on projects, and send in proof of your results. You can also go to Vermont to study with her in person or accompany Rosemary on one of her junkets to South America and other faraway places.

Other excellent courses are offered through Susan S. Weed at Wise Women Center, P.O. Box 64, Woodstock, NY 12498, through Hygieia College, P.O. Box 392, Monroe, UT 84754, and through Jeanne Rose at 219 Carl Street, San Francisco, CA 94117.

Years ago I took a course from Dominion Herbal College, 7427 Kingsway, Burnaby, BC V3N 3C1, Canada, and it helped me make the transition from Native American apprentice shaman to educated herbalist with a knowledge of botany and chemistry, as well as herbal medicine. The college's excellent reputation has been an important note on the résumé of many an alumni.

In Review

Much of the more comprehensive research I have utilized comes from a publication aimed at pharmacists and herbal practitioners called *The Lawrence Review of Natural Products*, which looks at specific herbs and other natural products each month in terms of their scientific and common names, botanical features, the history of their uses, pharmacology, and toxicology, and a summary of studies and experiments. Serious herbalists will want to get a subscription to this important research paper. The address is 111 West Port Plaza, Suite 400, St. Louis, MO 63146-3098.

Glossary

abortifacient: Causing or contributing to spontaneous abortion.

active principle: The component in a plant or substance that has a medicinal effect.

adaptogen: An agent that allows the body to adapt, particularly to stress.

adjuvant: A substance that aids or encourages the action of a treatment or medication.

alterative: This is usually a vague term for something that brings about change, but it is frequently encountered in older herbals, where it means a medium for renewal of the tissues.

amenorrhea: A spotty or suppressed menstrual discharge. *See* Dysmenorrhea.

analgesic: A pain reliever.

anesthetic: A numbing agent.

annual: A plant that lasts one year or season before dying.

Glossary

anodyne: Pain-easing.

anorectic: Lacking appetite.

anorexic: Causing loss of appetite.

anthelmintic: A treatment for intestinal parasites that kills or expels them from the body.

antibiotic: A substance that destroys germs or bacteria.

anticoagulant: A substance that prevents clotting.

antidiarrheal: Preventing loose stools.

antifungal: Inhibiting the growth of fungi.

antihemorrhagic: Curbing excessive blood flow and acting as a clotting agent.

antilithic: Working to treat or prevent kidney, gallbladder, or other calcium stones.

antioxidant: A substance that inhibits the formation of potentially dangerous toxins within the body. Antioxidants are thought to help prevent cancer and other chronic ailments.

antiperiodic: An agent that prevents recurrent fevers such as malaria.

antipruritic: An agent that prevents itching.

antipyretic: An agent that reduces fever.

antiscorbutic: Counteracting scurvy.

antiseptic: Preventing infection and killing germs.

antispasmodic: An agent that prevents spasms of muscles, nerves, or organs.

antitussive: Suppressing the cough reflex.

antiviral: Inhibiting the growth of a virus.

aperient: Any substance that promotes or induces natural movement of the bowels.

aphrodisiac: Having the power to excite the sexual organs or promote desire.

aromatic: An herb that smells or tastes good, or both. Aromatics are commonly used in cooking, but also are used to flavor mixtures made from other medicinal herbs that may be bitter or strong. Many aromatics also function as digestive aids. Common aromatics include allspice, anise, caraway, cardamom, cinnamon, clove, coriander, ginger, lemon peel, mint leaves, orange peel, sassafras, and vanilla bean. A simple medicine can be made with a 3:1:1 ratio using three parts of the medicinal herb, one part demulcent (*q.v.*), and one part aromatic. Some aromatics are themselves used as medicines.

astringent: An agent that causes the tissues to contract or bind.

bacillary: Of, relating to, or caused by a bacillus, a rod-shaped bacteria.

bitters: Substances that stimulate the appetite.

botánico: The Spanish word for herb doctor. A botánico may have either former medical training or knowledge passed down from one generation to the next, or both.

bruise: To break down the cells and release the medicinal oil in a plant's leaves by gently crushing them between your fingers, with a mortar and pestle, or between two rocks.

calmative: A substance that acts as a sedative.

carminative: Having the power to bring about the expulsion of gas and ease pains of the stomach and bowel.

catarrh: In the old days, this meant a cold or flulike syndrome. Today catarrh is defined as an inflammation of mucous membranes, usually including a fever or febrile condition.

cathartic: Producing strong evacuation of the bowels.

chilblains: An inflammatory swelling or sore caused by exposure to cold.

colic: Acute abdominal pain.

compress: A folded cloth or pad that is soaked in an herbal extract and then pressed on an inflamed or infected body part. Infusions, decoctions, and tinctures diluted with water can all be used to make a compress.

Glossary

cutaneous: Of or relating to the skin.

cystitis: See urinary tract infections

debridement: The surgical removal of damaged tissue.

decoction: An aqueous preparation obtained by vigorously boiling ingredients into a concentrated form. See chapter 2.

demulcent: An herb that possesses a soothing, usually mucilaginous
quality that relieves irritation to mucous membranes and other soft
tissues. Common demulcents include arrowroot, borage, coltsfoot,
licorice root, marshmallow leaves and root, oatmeal, okra pods,
sago root, sassafras pith, slippery elm bark, and Solomon's seal root.

diaphoretic: An agent that promotes sweating. Many diaphoretics also
increase metabolism and stimulate the body to increase temperature. Sweating is a healing technique used in some cultures.

diuretic: An agent that tends to increase the flow of urine. In general,
a diuretic allows the body to pass more fluids out than the ingested
amount. This principle is used in some weight-loss formulas and to
help treat water or fluid retention. Diuretics stimulate the kidneys.

double-blind study: A study in which neither the researchers nor the
subjects know who is receiving the medicine and who is receiving
a placebo.

dysemorrhea: Painful menstruation.

dyspepsia: Indigestion.

edema: Fluid retention, especially in the extremities, marked by
swelling and pain.

electrolytes: Bodily substances that conduct ions.

emesis: Vomiting.

emetic: A substance that causes vomiting.

emmenagogue: An agent that promotes menstruation.

emollient: Softening or soothing, especially to the skin.

enuresis: Involuntary discharge of urine; incontinence.

epistaxis: Nosebleed.

escapee: A plant (usually non-native) that once cultivated grows wild.

escharotic: An agent that causes a scab to form, which subsequently promotes healing.

expectorant: Loosening phlegm and aiding in expectoration or expulsion of phlegm. An agent that brings about a productive cough.

febrifuge: A substance that reduces fever.

febrile: Referring to fever, or increased body temperature.

galactagogue: An agent that induces or enhances the flow of milk.

gram negative and positive organism: Specific types of pathogens that require specific antibiotics to treat them.

halitosis: bad breath.

hepatic: Referring to the liver.

hypertension: High blood pressure.

hypnotic: Producing or bringing about sleep.

hypotension: Low blood pressure.

hypoxia: A deficiency of oxygen to the bodily tissues.

infusion: A preparation similar to tea, but stronger. An herb's active ingredients are released into water, which is then drunk. See chapter 2.

ischemia: Localized tissue anemia caused by an obstruction to the inflow of arterial blood.

jaundice: Yellowing of the skin, a sign of hepatitis or other liver problems. It is caused by the presence of bile pigments.

latex: Sap, usually milky and thick. In general, the term latex applies specifically to the sap of the rubber plant, but can also apply to other plants.

laxative: A bowel stimulant, bringing about bowel movement.

macerated: Originally this term meant "chewed," but it now refers to plant substances that have been softened in water or dissolved.

metate: A concave stone in which grain is ground into a powder or paste.

Glossary

mucilage: A gelatinous substance that protects mucous membranes and inflamed tissues.

mucilaginous: A soft, sticky, or slippery secretion or substance.

mucopolysaccharides: A substance found in bodily fluids and tissues that is made up of proteins and carbohydrates.

myasthenia gravis: A neuromuscular disease characterized by the progressive weakening and exhaustion of voluntary muscles.

myopia: Nearsightedness.

narcotic: Causing stupor and numbness.

nematicide: A preparation used to destroy parasitic worms.

nephritis: Acute or chronic inflammation of the kidney caused by infection, a degenerative process, or vascular disease.

nervine: A mild tranquilizer that restores or calms nerves.

neuralgia: Pain along a nerve.

ointment: An oil- or fat-based salve or unguent that is applied to the skin.

orexigenic: An appetite-stimulating substance.

oxytocic: Stimulating contractions of the womb.

parturifacient: An agent that induces or eases labor in childbirth.

parturition: The act of giving birth.

pectin: A substance that occurs naturally in apples and other fruits. When eaten, it prevents both diarrhea and constipation.

pectoral: Affecting the lungs and breathing.

perennial: A plant that grows or blossoms once a year, every year.

pertussis: Whooping cough.

phlebitis: Inflammation of a vein.

postparturient: Postpartum, referring to the period following childbirth.

poultice: A medicinal herbal paste that is applied to sores or lesions and then covered with a cloth.

prophylaxis: A measure designed to preserve good health and prevent the spread of disease.

Glossary

purgative: A synonym for "cathartic." A substance that tends to cause the body to expel unwanted or toxic substances. A purgative may work by means of elimination from the bowels or by emesis (vomiting).

refrigerant: A substance that relieves thirst or brings about cooling.

renal: Referring to the kidneys.

restorative: Something that serves to restore consciousness, vigor, or health.

rhizome: A subterranean plant stem that, unlike regular roots, produces buds, nodes, or scalelike leaves.

rubefacient: Any substance that causes reddening of the skin, usually affecting capillary blood flow. Sometimes it's a rub for muscular pain.

salve: An unctuous healing agent that is applied to wounds or sores.

sedative: Bringing about sleep, reducing nervous excitement.

silviculture: A branch of forestry dealing with the development and care of forests.

simple: An herb or medicine used on its own that does not produce any side effects.

sphagnum moss: The live green part of the peat moss plant, widely available at florists or in the wild.

sputum: Respiratory expectorant matter that contains saliva and other discharges.

stimulant: A substance that produces energy or activity.

stomachic: A drug that helps relieve stomach pain and cramping or reduces distention.

styptic: An externally applied substance to reduce bleeding.

sudorific: An agent that brings about copious sweating.

suspension: The state of a substance when its particles (e.g., a powder or clay) are mixed with but undissolved in a liquid, usually water; it must be shaken to maintain even distribution of the particles.

Glossary

synthesis: The combining of diverse elements into a coherent and unified whole.

systemic: Affecting the entire body.

taeniacide: A substance that kills tapeworms.

taeniafuge: An agent for expelling tapeworms from the body.

tannin: An astringent substance found in plants that is used in tanning, dyeing, and in the production of ink and medicine.

tincture: A medicinal solution in an alcohol base.

tonic: A substance that brings about a feeling of general well-being.

urticaria: Hives, itching, and inflammation of the skin caused by an allergic reaction.

vermifuge: A substance that expels worms from the body.

volunteer: A plant that grows spontaneously in a garden or elsewhere, often from a seed from a previous crop, or which is introduced by animals or accident.

vulnerary: Something that helps promote the healing of wounds.

wildcrafted: A plant that's harvested or gathered in the wild, as opposed to cultivated.

wort: Herb or plant.

Bibliography

Aikman, Lonelle. *Nature's Healing Arts.* Washington, D.C.: National Geographic Society, 1977.

Angier, Bradford P. *Field Guide to Medicinal Wild Plants.* Harrisburg, Pa.: Stackpole Books, 1978.

Blose, Nora, and Dawn Cusick. *Herb Drying Handbook.* New York: Sterling Publishing, 1993.

Brown, Tom. *Tom Brown's Guide to Wild Edible and Medicinal Plants.* New York: Berkley Books, 1985. And any of his other books.

Cairns, Huntington. *Shakespeare's Herbs.* Manteo, N.C.: The Elizabethan Gardens, 1984.

Castelman, Michael. *The Healing Herbs.* Emmaus, Pa.: Rodale Press, 1991.

Coon, Nelson. *Using Plants for Healing.* Emmaus, Pa.: Rodale Press, 1979.

Damian, Peter, and Kate Damian. *Aromatherapy: Scent and Psyche.* Rochester, Vt.: Healing Arts Press, 1995.

Bibliography

De La Tour, Shatoiya. *The Herbalist of Yarrow.* Sacramento, Calif.: Tzedakah Publications, 1994.

Duke, James A. *A CRC Handbook of Medicinal Herbs.* Boca Raton, Fla.: CRC Press, 1985.

———. *A Field Guide to Eastern and Central Medicinal Wild Plants.* New York: Houghton Mifflin, 1990.

———. *Handbook of Edible Weeds.* Boca Raton, Fla.: CRC Press, 1992.

———. *Handbook of Northeastern Indian Medicinal Plants.* Lincoln, Mass.: Quarterman Publications, 1986.

Elliot, Doug. *Wild Roots.* Rochester, Vt.: Healing Arts Press, 1995.

Foley, Denise, Eileen Nechas, and the editors of *Prevention* magazine. *Women's Encyclopedia of Health and Emotional Healing.* Emmaus, Pa.: Rodale Press, 1993.

Foster, Gertrude B., and Rosemary F. Louden. *Park's Success with Herbs.* Greenwood, S.C.: George W. Park Seed Co., 1980.

Flynn, Rebecca, and Mark Roest. *Your Guide to Standardized Herbs.* Prescott, Az.: One World Press, 1995.

Garrison, Robert, and Elizabeth Somer. *The Nutrition Desk Reference.* New Canaan, Conn.: Keats Publishing Co., 1995.

Gerard, John. *The Herball.* London, 1597; reprinted, New York: Dover Books, 1975.

Gibbons, Euell. *Stalking the Healthful Herbs.* Putney, Vt.: Alan C. Hood, 1966.

Gladstar, Rosemary. *Herbal Healing for Women.* New York: Simon & Schuster, 1993.

Green, James. *The Male Herbal.* Freedom, Calif.: Crossing Press, 1991.

Grieve, M. A. *A Modern Herbal.* 2 vols. Darien, Conn: Hafner Publishing Co., 1931; reprinted, New York: Dover Books, 1971 and 1982.

Bibliography

Harris, Ben Charles. *The Compleat Herbal*. New York: Bell Publishing Co., 1972.

Heinerman, John. *The Healing Benefit of Garlic*. New Canaan, Conn.: Keats Publishing, 1994.

Hsu, Hong-Yen, and William G. Preacher. *Chinese Herb Medicine and Therapy*. New Canaan, Conn.: Keats Publishing Co., 1982.

Hubbard, Mercer, with Julia Larke. *Anise to Woodruff*. Chapel Hill, N.C.: University of North Carolina Press, 1993.

Huson, Paul. *Mastering Herbalism*. New York: Stein & Day, 1974.

Hutchens, Alma R. *A Handbook of Native American Herbs*. Boston: Shambhala Publishers, 1992.

————. *Indian Herbalogy of North America*. Boston: Shambhala Publishers, 1991.

Jacobs, Betty E. M. *Growing and Using Herbs Successfully*. Pownal, Vt.: Garden Way Publishing, 1981.

King, Eleanor Anthony. *Bible Plants for American Gardens*. New York: Macmillan, 1941; reprinted, New York: Dover Books, 1975.

Kowalchick, Claire, and William H. Hylton, eds. *Rodale's Illustrated Encyclopedia of Herbs*. Emmaus, Pa.: Rodale Press, 1987.

Kloss, Jethro. *Back to Eden*. Loma Linda, Calif.: Back to Eden Books, 1981.

Kresanek, Jaraslav. *Healing Plants*. New York: Arco Publishing, 1985.

Krochmal, Arnold, and Connie Krochmal. *A Field Guide to Medicinal Plants*. New York: Times Books, 1984.

Leung, Albert Y. *Chinese Herbal Remedies*. New York: Universe Books, 1984.

Lust, John. *The Herb Book*. New York: Benedict Lust Publications, 1974.

Mann. Charles C., and Mark L. Plummer. *The Aspirin Wars*. New York: Alfred A. Knopf, 1991.

Bibliography

Martinez, Jose R. *Yerbario Medicinal Mexicano.* San Miguel, Mexico: Editores Mexicanos Unidos, S.A., 1983.

Matthews, Doris J. *Old Fashioned Herbs for Modern Living.* Nashville, Tenn.: Sparrow Hill, 1983.

McBride, L. R. *Practical Folk Medicine of Hawaii.* Hilo, Hawaii: Petroglyph Press, 1975.

Mellinger, Marie. *Roadside Rambles.* Tiger, Ga.: self-published, n.d.

Meyer, Joseph. *The Herbalist.* Glenwood, Ill.: Meyerbooks, 1918, 1986.

Mills, Simon Y. *Out of the Earth.* New York: Penguin Books, 1991.

Millspaugh, Charles F. *American Herbal Plants.* n.p. 1892; reprinted, New York: Dover Books, 1974.

Mindell, Earl. *Earl Mindell's Herb Bible.* New York: Simon & Schuster, 1992.

Mowrey, Daniel B. *The Scientific Validation of Herbal Medicine.* New York: Cormorant Books, 1986.

Murray, Michael T. *The Healing Power of Herbs.* Rocklin, Calif.: Prima Publishing, 1992.

Parvati, Jeannine. *Hygieia: A Woman's Herbal.* Berkeley, Calif.: Freestone Books, 1978.

Persons, W. Scott. *American Ginseng: Green Gold.* Asheville, N.C.: Bright Mountain Books, 1994.

Peterson, Lee Allen. *A Field Guide to Edible Wild Plants.* New York: Houghton Mifflin, 1977.

Pond, Barbara. *A Sampler of Wayside Herbs.* New York: Greenwich House, 1974.

Prevention magazine, editors. *The Doctor's Book of Home Remedies.* Emmaus, Pa.: Rodale Press, 1990.

Reader's Digest. *Magic and Medicine of Plants.* Pleasantville, N.Y.: Reader's Digest Association, 1986.

Reppert, Bertha. *Growing Your Own Herb Business.* Pownal, Vt.: Storey Communications, 1994.

Romm, Aviva Jill. *Natural Healing for Babies and Children.* Freedom, Calif.: Crossing Press, 1996.

Scott, Michael B. *An Irish Herbal.* Wellingborough, U.K.: Aquarian Press, 1986.

Simmons, Adelma G. *Herb Gardens of Delight.* Tolland, Conn.: Clinton Press, 1974.

―――. *Herbs to Grow Indoors.* New York: Hawthorn Books, 1969.

Squier, Thomas K. *The Wild and Free Cookbook.* Port Townsend, Wash.: Loompanics Unlimited, 1996.

Stark, Debra. *Round-the-World-Cooking at the Natural Gourmet.* New Canaan, Conn.: Keats Publishing, 1994.

Stein, Diane. *The Natural Remedy Book for Dogs and Cats.* Freedom, Calif.: Crossing Press, 1994.

Sturdivant, Lee. *Herbs for Sale.* Friday Harbor, Wash.: San Juan Naturals, 1994.

―――. *Profits from Your Backyard Herb Garden.* Friday Harbor, Wash.: San Juan Naturals, 1988.

Tierra, Michael, ed. *American Herbalism.* Freedom, Calif.: Crossing Press, 1992.

Torres, Eliseo. *Green Medicine.* Kingsville, Texas: Nieves Press, n.d.

Tyler, Varro E. *Herbs of Choice.* Binghamton, N.Y.: Pharmaceutical Products Press, 1994.

―――. *The Honest Herbal.* Binghamton, N.Y.: Pharmaceutical Products Press, 1993.

Vogel, Virgil J. *American Indian Medicine.* Norman, Okla.: University of Oklahoma Press, 1970.

Walking, Night Bear, and Stan Padilla. *Song of the Seven Herbs.* Summertown, Tenn.: Book Publishing Co., 1983.

Weil, Andrew. *The Marriage of Sun and Moon.* New York: Houghton Mifflin, 1980.

Weiner, Michael. *Earth Medicine, Earth Food.* New York: Macmillan, 1980.

Bibliography

Wilbur, C. Keith. *Revolutionary Medicine.* Old Saybrook, Conn.: Globe
    Pequot Press, 1980.
Wood, Edelene. *A Taste of the Wild.* Elgin, Pa.: Allegheny Press, 1990.
Wren, R. C. *Potter's New Cyclopedia of Botanical Drugs and Preparations.*
    Essex, U.K.: 1907; reprinted, Essex, U.K.: C. W. Daniel Co., Ltd.,
    1988.

THOMAS BROKEN BEAR SQUIER is a licensed Naturopath in his home state of North Carolina, writer, lecturer, and a regular columnist for *The Fayetteville Observer-Times*. He received his initial training in herbal medicine from his grandfather, a self-educated Cherokee root doctor. During his tenure as a Green Beret he taught survival training and helped the army revise its field manual. He is also the author of *Living Off the Land Wild Foods Cookbook*. He lives with his family in North Carolina, where he also serves as a Veteran Services Officer.